MINDSTORMS

MINDSTORMS

The Complete Guide for Families Living with Traumatic Brain Injury

John W. Cassidy, M.D.

with Karla Dougherty

Da Capo
∞
LIFE
LONG

A MEMBER OF THE
PERSEUS BOOKS GROUP

Copyright © 2009 by John W. Cassidy, M.D.
Illustrations © 2009 by Neal Rohrer

Set in 11 point Palatino by the Perseus Books Group

Library of Congress Cataloging-in-Publication Data
Cassidy, John W.
  Mindstorms : the complete guide for families living with traumatic brain injury / John W. Cassidy.
     p. cm.
  Includes index.
  ISBN 978-0-7382-1247-0 (alk. paper)
  1. Brain—Wounds and injuries—Complications. 2. Brain—Wounds and injuries—Patients—Rehabilitation. 3. Brain damage. I. Title.
  RD594.C37 2009
  617.4'81044—dc22

                              2008038637

First Da Capo Press edition 2009

Published by Da Capo Press
A Member of the Perseus Books Group
www.dacapopress.com

Note: The information in this book is true and complete to the best of our knowledge. This book is intended only as an informative guide for those wishing to know more about health issues. In no way is this book intended to replace, countermand, or conflict with the advice given to you by your own physician. The ultimate decision concerning care should be made between you and your doctor. We strongly recommend you follow his or her advice. Information in this book is general and is offered with no guarantees on the part of the author or Da Capo Press. The author and publisher disclaim all liability in connection with the use of this book. Nearly all of the names and identifying details of people associated with events described in this book have been changed. Any similarity to actual persons is coincidental.

10 9 8 7 6 5 4 3 2 1

This book is dedicated to those who took the leap of faith:

RAYMOND D. ADAMS, MD; CHARLENE MADISON CASSIDY, PHD;
BRUCE M. COHEN, MD, PHD; SHERVERT FRAZIER, MD;
AND NORMAN A. ZOBER, PHD.

CONTENTS

PART 4

THE JOURNEY BACK

FOREWORD

A brain injury is a life-altering experience. For some, the changes are subtle, hidden. For others, the differences can be more dramatic, causing alterations in personality, thought, and movement that are permanent.

Most brain injuries happen in seconds: a car accident, a stroke or aneurism, a fall or sports injury. In my family's case it was a bomb on a dusty road in Iraq.

My husband, Bob Woodruff, an anchor of ABC News, was embedded with the military near Baghdad during the Iraq War in 2006. While he was standing in a tank, but with his head exposed through a hatch, a remote-controlled 155 mm shell exploded at close range. The force of the blast and the shrapnel blew off Bob's helmet and crushed his left temporal lobe, also injuring the left side of his face and neck.

In an instant our lives became focused solely on Bob's survival as he lay in a coma for thirty-six days, battling back from the injury and then succumbing to sepsis and pneumonia following numerous surgeries. Like so many before me I became a full-time caregiver, balancing my children's needs against those of my husband and praying, hoping, believing that he would have a good outcome, despite the grim prognosis. During this time, I became determined to get as much information as I could.

For anyone involved—whether patients or their loved ones—navigating the journey of brain injury can be frightening, complex, and often discouraging. There are far too few beacons of information, hope, and realism. I

1

initially picked up the manuscript of this book expecting to find something geared more to professionals, something that would speak in mostly inaccessible language and foreign terminology.

What I found instead was a breath of fresh air among the many other publications I have seen. *Mindstorms* is a useful, interesting, and informative manual, almost breezy in its comfortable ability to communicate with the layperson. I read it cover to cover. One of the greatest gifts you can be handed in the midst of a storm is a life raft. This book is that raft. It offers families one comprehensive place to access all the information, knowledge, and answers to common questions they will need by laying out easy-to-follow examples, explanations, stories, analogies, and even diagrams.

This book accomplishes something very difficult—it demystifies the most complex and individual organ in our bodies. And it does so in a tone that is not overly cheerful, full of doom and gloom, or patronizing. Above all, I found that to be comforting.

We will never be able to eradicate brain injuries from humanity. There will always be accidents, injuries, violence, and the unpredictability of life. But one thing that can ease the journey is a book like this, offering some good sense out of what is often, especially initially, a senseless situation.

—Lee Woodruff, coauthor with Bob Woodruff of
In An Instant: A Family's Journey of Love and Healing

INTRODUCTION

Jessica Collins, a professional aerobics instructor who worked out six times a week, had been married to Kyle for a year and still felt like a newlywed. Around noon on a hot August day, she was on her way in her sports coupe to meet Kyle for lunch.

And then her life changed forever.

A pickup truck going seventy miles per hour hit her car broadside on the driver's side, knocking Jessica unconscious. She was rushed to the hospital with serious internal injuries, including a damaged spleen, a broken collarbone, and a massive brain injury that affected both sides of her brain.

"I'll never forget that day as long as I live," said Jessica's mother, Laura. "I lived two hours away and had just registered to go back to college. Kyle's mother called me with the news, and I was in the car before we even hung up."

So many family members gathered at the hospital that one of the doctors let them wait in an empty conference room. Finally, a doctor came in and said, "I want to talk to y'all. I'll bring you in to see Jessica now, but you have to be prepared for what you're going to see. She may be unconscious for the rest of her life. She may never talk again."

Hours later, Jessica's brain began to swell up so much that a neurosurgeon had to drill two burr holes in her skull to relieve the elevated pressure. She was put into a deep coma with medications to give her brain a chance to heal. Although the doctors kept telling the family to prepare for the worst, Laura tried to focus on any positive sign, no matter how slight. If Jessica blinked, it was an improvement. If Jessica moved her head a millimeter at the sound of her mom's voice, it was progress.

"Enough, Jessica," Laura would whisper to her. "I've had it. Time for you to wake up. You have a strong body. I know you do. Tell your brain that this is what is going to happen: You are going to be Jessica again."

Slowly, very slowly, Jessica began her journey back. After a three-and-a-half-month stay—first at the trauma center, and then at a long-term specialty medical hospital—she was transferred to a rehabilitation facility, where she relearned basic routines, such as taking a shower, brushing her teeth, getting dressed, going by herself to the bathroom. Once she had these activities of daily living down, she was discharged, but she remained an outpatient for a year. Her biggest fear was that she would never have children.

Jessica couldn't remember the accident then and never will. In fact, she couldn't remember anything further back than her last birthday, a month before the accident. Laura began writing in a journal about Jessica's life before and after the traumatic brain injury, so that even if she couldn't remember the events, at least she would have a record of them.

Today, Jessica works out every other day in her home gym, lifting weights and riding a stationary bike. She has two children, who, she says, are perfect (of course!). She loves to read Danielle Steele novels, and her mother drives her to the day-care center her daughter Haley attends, where Jessica works with other children part-time as a classroom aide.

Is Jessica the same person she was before the accident? No. She slurs her words when she gets nervous or tired. She drops things and has difficulty moving around in crowds. She still has short-term memory issues and can't drive a car. But Jessica has accepted her new life with its limitations. She is surrounded by love, and that makes up for a lot.

Jessica's tragedy is one of thousands that occur each year—each one as unique as the person involved. Traumatic brain injuries are always caused by a number of pathologic changes to the brain, depending on the type or types of injuries involved in the initial trauma. In medical terms, these pathologic changes are referred to as the *underlying neuropathology*. Some of these end results of trauma are caused by the same neuropathology that afflicts individuals who have experienced non-trauma-related disorders such as strokes, heart attacks *(myocardial infarctions)*, or near-drowning.

For example, strokes that result from abnormalities occurring in the blood vessels supplying the brain with blood and oxygen are caused either by blockage or rupture of these blood vessels. Although under these circumstances the pathologic processes that impact brain functioning are not generally related to trauma, stroke-like syndromes are commonly seen following traumatic brain injuries when these same vessels are injured by externally produced forces that tear or compress them. Similarly, heart attacks or near drowning lead to deprivation of oxygen and blood flow to the entire brain. In the case of a full-blown cardiopulmonary arrest, the heart is unable to pump blood; in the case of near drowning, the lungs fill with water and prevent oxygen from reaching the brain. These conditions cause either hypoxemia or anoxia, which destroys large areas of brain cells when they do not receive enough *(hypoxemia)* or any *(anoxia)* oxygen for periods of five to ten minutes. After ten to twelve minutes without oxygen, most people cannot survive. In cases of traumatic brain injury, such oxygen deprivation can be produced by massive internal bleeding from damage to a patient's abdominal organs or severe blood loss associated with broken bones in the legs.

BY THE NUMBERS

Did you know that a brain injury occurs every twenty seconds in the United States? Over 1 million of these brain-injured people are rushed to hospital emergency rooms and trauma centers every year.

Even more sobering, Jessica, described above, is just one of an estimated 6.3 million Americans (2 percent of the population) who live with a severe disability caused by traumatic brain injury (TBI). In 2008 alone, there were 1.6 million cases of brain injury caused by direct trauma to the brain.

Brain injuries are more common in the United States than such conditions as breast cancer, AIDS, multiple sclerosis, and spinal cord injury. The number of people surviving falls, strokes, and military or gang-related injuries has grown, and, as a result, there are more brain-injured survivors than ever before. Yet, despite these numbers, most Americans think of brain injury as one of those rare events in life. In fact, those who are aware of its prevalence have often referred to it as a silent epidemic.

If you have picked up this book, you are probably either someone who has suffered a brain injury yourself or a caregiver for someone with such an injury. These numbers should help you understand that brain injury isn't so rare. That awareness can help you to realize that you are not alone.

THE EFFECTS OF BRAIN INJURY

Brain damage typically occurs as a result of a fall, a car accident, a stroke, a heart attack, an explosion, or a gunshot wound to the head. With any luck, the damage is mild and the victim will be as good as new in just a few months. In other cases, it may be more severe, the result of vital oxygen being withheld from the brain cells, increased pressure on the brain due to internal damage, or bruising caused by the movement of the brain within the ridges of the skull. Some of the most debilitating symptoms of brain injury may not become apparent for days, weeks, or even months after the event. And typically those symptoms involve a person's memories and behavior.

When you have a heart attack, your heart can lose its capacity to pump blood throughout your system. When you have congestion in your lungs, you may have difficulty breathing. Thus, it makes sense that when you hurt your brain—the organ of the mind—*it may affect your behavior.*

As simple as this concept is, many people have a hard time accepting it. Changes in behavior scare people. If someone you love has suffered a brain injury, that person you knew so well may suddenly seem like a stranger— someone who doesn't act the same way, doesn't think the same way, and who may even become violent or not remember your name.

The particular symptoms vary from individual to individual. I, as a doctor, can say that if the brain is damaged in the frontal lobe—the area closest to the forehead—the patient will most likely have difficulty in organizing thoughts, making basic plans, or carrying out basic routines in sequential order. But I can't say *exactly* how that change will manifest itself. One person may dry himself off *before* taking his shower. Another may ask the same question over and over again, unable to understand the answer. Yet another will have difficulty carrying out the most basic tasks, such as making a sandwich or doing laundry. And still another person may shout curses at the top of his lungs.

I can say that if the areas near the temples, the temporal lobes, are also damaged, it may affect memory. But I can't say exactly how that will happen. One person may remember the song "Happy Birthday" but look at you blankly if you mention something from the nightly news you both just watched. Another person may recognize the image of her mother, but be unable to say her name.

I can also say that a brain injury may create physical impairments, from partial paralysis to lack of coordination. It can cause problems in basic human functions, from the ability to swallow to knowing when to go to the bathroom. But I can't say exactly how these problems—physical, cognitive, or emotional—will play out.

Nor can I say with certainty to what extent a patient will recover. We know that early intervention can help stave off the worst TBI symptoms. We also know that the brain itself will try to adapt, creating new passageways to circumvent the damage. We know the brain can be retrained to remember, to organize, to keep emotions in check. And we know that the more severe the injury, the slower and more difficult the recovery will be. But, once again, we don't know the specifics of how any individual will heal or not heal.

In short, the experiences that have nurtured, sustained, and created a particular personality throughout the years have created patterns in the brain that are unique to that individual. And if the brain is damaged, the individual's behavior—physical, cognitive, and emotional—will be affected. The specifics of the behavior changes, however, will vary from person to person.

THE ALIEN SELF

There is no greater nightmare than waking up and discovering that the self you took for granted is gone. From *A Beautiful Mind* to *The Bourne Identity,* the loss of self has been the theme behind many a classic Hollywood movie. But what makes TBI even more painful and difficult to deal with is that often its victims are biologically unable to realize that they are different and have residual disabilities. However, the parent, spouse, friend, or lover will know beyond a shadow of a doubt. Both victim and supporter are joined together in an extremely unusual and complex pain. Together, you must make the difficult journey back to a functioning family, to fulfilling friendships, and to productive activity that are the hallmarks of a successful rehabilitation.

When I was working on my residency at various Harvard Medical School training hospitals, my neurology colleagues always sent me the patients who showed emotional and behavioral damage; they were able to handle physical symptoms, but the uncharted territory of the "alien self" left them cold. At the same time, my psychiatry colleagues always sent me their "worst case" patients—the ones with such extensive brain injury that my colleagues had given up on trying to repair their fragile egos.

I'm grateful to these long-ago colleagues. It was helping these so-called hopeless cases rediscover those things we undamaged people take for granted, those very things that make us human, that fed my passion and gave me back a thousandfold what I gave them. With over twenty-five years of experience helping TBI patients, I can now say with certainty that proper treatment *can* make a difference—if not for the patients, then for the loved ones who must take care of them, day in and day out.

It isn't fast. It isn't easy. But it isn't impossible.

YOU ARE IN GOOD COMPANY

As you read, you will meet some wonderful people who have suffered, and continue to live with, brain injury. I am honored that they have been willing to share their stories with me. These are people just like you and me, but with one profound difference: They all had a brain injury and survived. As a result, life irrevocably changed for them and their loved ones. But as their stories unfold you'll find that there is life after brain injury, and that hope never dies.

Emily Carter sustained a severe traumatic brain injury as a result of a car accident in icy weather in 1992. She was eighteen years old at the time and had dreams of completing college and becoming a broadcaster, marrying, and having children. Within seconds, when her car skidded on an icy road and ran into the path of oncoming traffic, all that changed. Her fight for re-covery has, as of this writing, involved fifteen years of daily work to over-come the disabilities that once threatened her independence and the realization of all her dreams. The intensely difficult work she had to do when first hospitalized has paid off. She still uses many of the strategies that she used to relearn to speak intelligibly, walk safely on uneven sur-faces, and independently dress herself. Later, she also had to overcome dangerous impulsivity and severe depression. In one of our recent sessions, she told me she finally liked this new Emily even better than the old one!

John Stambino was an up-and-coming musician in 2000. He and his band were scheduled to play a gig at a club in downtown Manhattan, but they never got there. They stopped at a convenience store, where a stranger shot John and one of his band members, along with five other people, and then killed himself. John's friend didn't survive, and John had most of the frontal portion of his brain destroyed. Eventually, he regained the ability to walk and speak, but he has posttraumatic epilepsy that requires daily use of antiseizure medications and close monitoring. However, he struggles with coming to terms with the fact that he is different. He tried returning to the stage. He had one great night, then he found that the strobe lights caused him to have severe seizures. Now, he is forging a new life, working part-time at a food bank near his Connecticut home and playing guitar with his friends on the weekends.

Y. J. Ming went jogging early one morning in 1993 in New York City. While running, he suddenly fell to the ground. The cause? A cardiac arrest caused by an abnormal heart rhythm that stopped the flow of oxygen to his brain for more than five minutes, leading to a full-blown cardiopulmonary arrest. Fortunately, some bystanders were able to perform CPR on him. Despite their efforts, he sustained a very serious type of acquired brain injury referred to as anoxic brain injury. It left him with, among other symptoms, severe short-term memory deficits, despite the fact that he looked perfectly normal when he left the hospital. Prior to the heart attack, he had been a high-powered Wall Street executive. Today, although unable to work—because he still has considerable short-term memory deficits—he has found a way to be a productive member of his community and church. He and his wife, Mia, have two wonderful kids who have adapted themselves to their dad's limitations.

Sam O'Connell, a marine stationed in Iraq, was planning his homecoming in two weeks. After a brief stay outside Baghdad, he was in a Humvee returning to his base camp with five of his buddies when tragedy struck. They drove over an improvised explosive device (IED), and their Humvee was blown into the air. Sam, who'd been sitting in the back, was ejected from the vehicle at the time of first impact. His buddies weren't as fortunate. Sam came home to Pennsylvania a hero, but a reluctant one. He kept thinking about his fellow marines who hadn't made it home. He couldn't sleep, and his mind kept flashing back to that day of the explosion. After several months, it became clear that despite a mild brain injury with some postconcussive symptoms, his major problem was posttraumatic stress disorder. His symptoms worsened to the point where he stopped getting out of bed in the morning. At that point, he needed, and did receive, professional help.

Louise McDougal was her high school's head cheerleader during her senior year. One of the most exciting formations their group performed was a human pyramid, with Louise leaping to the top position at the grand finale. However, during the homecoming game, a teammate's ankle gave out, and Louise fell, fracturing her skull but not losing consciousness. Because initially she only felt shook up, she continued cheering for the next ten minutes. However, she then collapsed into a coma and was rushed to the emergency room. A ruptured artery was discovered as a result of her skull fracture, and immediate surgery was required. Her road to recovery took well over a year as she underwent intensive inpatient treatment at a specialty medical hospital. Although she returned home, her parents had to cope with the fact that they had lost the Louise they had known up until then.

Troy Atkins was sixteen when he suffered his brain injury. An Olympic-caliber marksman, he was skeet shooting with his father when his rifle, for some reason, exploded. As the shot was fired, the top part of the barrel flipped up, hit him in the head, and became embedded there. A neurosurgeon had to cut a hole around the barrel and into his brain to carefully remove fragments that had become lodged in the brain tissue. The force of the injury led to a significant increase in the pressure on his brain, and during the surgery, a monitor was placed to continuously check the pressure of his swelling brain. He had bruising and bleeding in the layers of tissue between his brain and the inside of his skull. Because Troy's injury was more localized than diffuse, his recovery was significantly better than might have been expected. Today he is in college, but he requires special accommodations at school in order to successfully complete his classes.

These are only a few of the people who have survived brain injuries. Each one is unique, and so the strategies used to help them had to be customized to their particular needs and individual strengths and weaknesses. Time and team-oriented quality care have helped. So have the love and support that family and friends have offered along the journey to recovery. As you read through this book, think of these people—how they have survived and forged a new life, despite what happened to them. It is my sincere hope their stories will help you get through your own unique mindstorm.

WHAT TO EXPECT FROM THIS BOOK

In what follows, I have attempted to strike a balance between becoming too technical, on the one hand, and oversimplifying the material, on the other. I strove to present information in a way that is understandable to those encountering these concepts for the first time. I encourage you to use this book as it best suits you, either by reading it from start to finish or by dipping into those sections that seem most relevant to you at the moment.

In Part 1, I lay the foundation for understanding brain injury by identifying the basic types of injury and explaining how various types are classified and diagnosed. (For those looking for a more detailed explanation of the way the brain works or wanting specific definitions, please consult the appendix.) I also explore some myths that still surround both the brain and the injuries that affect it in order to help correct the distortions popularized by forms of entertainment such as TV shows and movies, with specific attention to the return of consciousness following coma. This section ends with a discussion of mild traumatic brain injury (MTBI), the most common type of traumatic injury to the brain occurring within the general population.

In Part 2, I focus on the ways in which a brain injury impacts the body, the mind, the social behavior, and the personality of the individual it afflicts.

In Part 3, I look at the treatment provided to brain-injured patients, starting from their arrival in the emergency room, including surgery, if needed. I also cover the common medications used in the treatment of TBI and various types of physical, cognitive, and behavioral therapies. The choice of therapeutic intervention depends on the severity of the injuries and the residual deficits that remain. Contemporary interdisciplinary neurorehabilitation is discussed with a focus on limiting handicapping conditions, reducing the burden of caring for those with severe injuries, and limiting the behavioral and memory issues that become most problematic for survivors and their families as time progresses.

Finally, in Part 4, the focus is on the process of reentering the real world as a patient leaves formal rehabilitative treatment, returns home, and begins to work again or attend school. I conclude with some thoughts for the caregivers of those who have been injured to help them cope with the demands of their important role. When one member of a family sustains a brain injury, the treatment and rehabilitative process inevitably becomes a family affair.

My primary goal in writing this book is to provide information placed in its proper context based on my experience in caring for brain-injured patients and their families for many years. "Information," such as that supplied by well-meaning friends or Internet sites, is never a substitute for real knowledge that comes from wisdom gained through experience.

Brain injury remains a silent epidemic a decade after the U.S. Congress heralded the 1990s as the "the decade of the brain." In writing this book I was also committed to another goal: getting the word out about the sobering realities that many people face because of a lack of comprehensive knowledge among members of the general public about the impact of traumatic brain injury on the lives of so many people. I hope this awareness will mobilize all of us to continue to work toward the prevention of traumatic brain injuries and to promote continued research into new theories that may ultimately lead to their cure.

Perhaps most compelling, in the pages to come you will find the stories of many people who have suffered through TBI, either as survivors or caregivers. You will journey with them through the life-changing impact of their accidents; you will be with them as they cope with their TBI symptoms; you will experience the joy of their reentry into the world. Whether you are a TBI survivor or a caregiver, you will find experiences that echo yours in their stories. I expect you will be inspired by their journeys and gain strength from their newfound lives. And, more than anything else, you will realize you are not alone.

I hope this book will inspire you along with all caregivers and survivors dealing with MTBI or TBI and that it will help to take you to that final frontier, where a better quality of life awaits both of you, where dignity goes both ways, and where you understand that good, solid care starts with yourself.

Along with the many heroic survivors whom I have had the privilege to treat over these many years, this book is also dedicated to the caregivers, those of you who are living with and recovering from the shock, and, in some cases, the irrevocable changes, that come when a loved one suffers from a brain trauma. I hope to provide insight, education, and relief from the pain, the guilt, and the daily grind that you, the caregiver, must carry. And by helping you, this book will also give your brain-injured loved one the help he needs, the care she so deserves.

This book contains information that no caregiver should be without. Over the past ten years, extensive new knowledge has been gained about the brain and how it works, as well as about brain injury recovery and rehabilitation. There have been changes in the way we diagnose brain injury and view its damage. *Mindstorms* is my attempt to provide not only compassion but education. In knowledge, there is strength—for everyone.

PART 1

UNDERSTANDING THE BASICS OF BRAIN INJURY

chapter 1

Types of Traumatic Brain Injury

> *I had a really serious head injury. I don't know*
> *the meaning of any of this. I don't know the*
> *whys and wherefores.*
>
> —Barbara Mandrell

In 2006, *ABC-TV Evening News* anchor Bob Woodruff was covering the Iraq War, embedded with the Fourth Infantry Division. Although he normally interviewed American soldiers, he wanted to get a story from the Iraqi perspective. He was riding in an Iraqi tank when a shell detonated in the road; the explosion blew through the left side of his head and ripped open his neck. He nearly bled to death in the tank as the battle raged on around him. Fortunately, he was rapidly extracted by American forces and taken to a nearby medical base where he underwent eight hours of surgery to stop the bleeding and remove the debris from his head and neck. Still, the explosive force, as well as the flying shrapnel, caused extensive brain damage. He had a remarkable recovery, and today his major difficulty is finding the right words to express himself. A year later, he and his wife, Lee, wrote *In an Instant*, a best-selling memoir about his TBI experience and how it affected his whole family. They also have established a foundation to raise money to help other TBI victims.

James Brady is another of the most influential—and inspiring—people with traumatic brain injury living today. During a 1981 assassination attempt on then–president Ronald Reagan, he caught a bullet to his head and fell to the ground, unconscious. He survived but was left paralyzed, and remains wheelchair-bound to this day. Rather than become just another statistic, he began advocating for gun control and along with his wife, Sarah, established the Brady Center to Prevent Gun Violence. They saw the fruits of their labor in 1993 when the Brady Handgun Violence Prevention Act, dubbed the "Brady Bill," became law. In 1996, he received the Presidential Medal of Freedom, the highest honor a civilian can earn for service to his country.

In 1994, legendary NASCAR driver Ernie Irvan (a.k.a. "Swerving Irvan") crashed into a wall during a practice session while traveling at a speed of over 170 miles per hour. He suffered extensive brain damage and was given a 10 percent chance for survival. A few weeks after the accident, he was transferred to a rehabilitation hospital, and less than two months later he appeared in person to receive a NASCAR award in New York. He continued to work hard on his rehabilitation, but five years later he once again crashed during a practice session and suffered another brain injury. This time, he had to retire and hang up his "wheels."

Patricia Neal was the Nicole Kidman of her day. She appeared in many highly acclaimed movies, including *The Subject Was Roses* and *The Fountainhead*, as well as Broadway shows such as *The Miracle Worker*. In 1965, while she was pregnant, she suffered a stroke. Neal was in a coma for three weeks, and when she regained consciousness, she couldn't walk or talk, let alone act. But through determination, a bit of luck, and the devotion of her family, she made an amazing comeback. Her comment at the time: "I'm just stubborn, that's all."

Called the Princess of Steel because of her way with a steel guitar, country singer Barbara Mandrell was at the top of her game in the 1970s and early 1980s, noted for the classic song "I Was Country Before Country Was Even Cool." But in 1984, a driver swerved into her lane on a highway and hit her car head-on. Luckily, her children escaped serious injury, but Barbara suffered multiple fractures and bruises and sustained a severe head injury that left her depressed for a year. Eventually, however, she reemerged on the country music scene with a vengeance with hits like

SOBERING STATISTICS

- Approximately 1.6 million people have a traumatic brain injury every year, more than triple the number of people who get breast cancer.
- More than 6.3 million Americans live with a TBI disability.
- Falls are the leading cause of TBI (28 percent). Second place goes to car and other motor vehicle accidents (20 percent).
- 80,000 to 90,000 people per year suffer long-term disabilities after a TBI.
- Men are 1.5 to 2 times more likely to get a TBI than women.
- The two age groups most at risk are young children (from birth to age four) and teens (ages fifteen to nineteen).
- African Americans have the highest rate of death after a TBI.
- TBI costs Americans over $56.3 billion every year.
- As of 2007, more than 80,000 veterans of the Iraq and Afghanistan wars have been discharged because of medical conditions "affecting the nervous system."

"Angel in Your Arms" and "Get to the Heart." She also started acting on television and wrote a best-selling book about her life. These celebrities have risen above their brain injuries to become inspiring role models for others. They worked hard in the months—and years—of rehabilitation and recovery to survive as intact as possible, and some have resumed successful careers.

Although rehabilitation treatment varies from person to person, recovery depends on both the type and the severity of brain injury as well as the brain's ability to heal, adapt, and compensate for residual deficits that may last a lifetime.

THE BIG FOUR

There are four major types of brain injury: focal contusional injury; focal hemorrhagic or ischemic injury; diffuse axonal injury; and diffuse hypoxemic or anoxic injury. My intention in outlining these different types of brain injury is not to scare you, but rather to help explain exactly what these technical terms that you may have heard in the doctor's office mean. All four types may occur as a result of a single event. Let's take a brief look at each one.

Focal Contusional Injury

The first type, *focal contusional injury,* refers to bruising of specific areas of the brain as a result of abrasion by the boney, roughened skull. Contusions are often associated with tears in the brain tissue *(lacerations)* that can cause bleeding or swelling in the brain. This bruising is termed *focal* because it occurs in specific areas of the brain rather than generally throughout the entire brain. Thus, these injuries are far more common in areas of the brain that come into contact with roughed areas of the skull in the front of the brain (behind the forehead and above the eyes) and at its sides at the level of the ears. The brain can be damaged at the point of direct impact, as well as on the opposite side of the impact, by the striking that occurs on the inside of the skull during the traumatic event. When this occurs, it is called a *coup-contrecoup injury.*

Focal Hemorrhagic, or Ischemic, Injury

The second type of injury, *focal ischemic or hemorrhagic injury,* is caused by blockage or rupture of specific blood vessels that supply certain areas of the brain with oxygen. This type of damage is common in stroke (which is discussed in greater detail later in this chapter) but often occurs in traumatic brain injuries as well. Describing these injuries as *focal* emphasizes that they are localized to specific areas of the brain. (Injuries affecting the entire brain are termed *diffuse.)* The results of these injuries depend on what area of the brain was supplied by the now blocked or ruptured blood vessels *(arteries* and *veins),* as well as the size of the area of cell death. In ischemic injuries, areas of the brain are damaged by the deprivation of blood and oxygen supply. Hemorrhagic injuries occur when blood vessels rupture and produce both bleeding in the brain and loss of supply to areas of the brain normally supplied by the burst vessels. Brain cells *(neurons)* cannot survive more than six or seven minutes without oxygenated blood,

NOT ALL HEAD INJURIES CAUSE BRAIN INJURIES

Although the terms are sometimes used interchangeably, there is a difference between a head injury and a brain injury. We've all hit our heads without "blacking out," and it can hurt—a lot. But a few cold compresses later, you're out and about with nothing more than a little lump. That's a **head injury.**

A **brain injury,** however, is an injury to the brain itself. Its effects are far more serious. Brain injury can occur from an impact to the head or from violent shaking of the head (such as occurs in what is known as "shaken baby syndrome"). The head may look fine, but there's damage that can't be seen—bleeding, swelling, malfunction—within the brain.

so death of these cells occurs very rapidly. Given this localization, one person may be unable to speak, another unable to move his arm or leg, for example.

Other mechanisms may produce the same effect by compressing specific areas of the brain or pushing parts of it into spaces where there is no room for it. As an example, direct trauma to the skull may produce a skull fracture that ruptures a major artery supplying oxygen to the coverings of the brain. This leads to massive, rapid bleeding in the area between the skull and the brain, a condition called an *epidural hematoma* (a local collection of blood); within minutes, it can become life-threatening by pushing the incompressible brain into areas within the skull and the nearby areas surrounding the brain stem and spinal column that cannot accommodate these structures. Unless this hemorrhage is rapidly stopped with surgery, this severe displacement of the brain will likely cause death.

Diffuse Axonal Injury

The third type of brain injury affects the entire brain and is referred to as *diffuse axonal injury (DAI)*. It occurs when the brain is shaken and remains in motion inside the skull as it decelerates more slowly than the skull. The brain actually bounces around inside the skull, its nerve cells being pulled, stretched, and torn like elastic bands. Since the forces involved also include rotation of the head around the neck, the entire brain is impacted by this diffuse form of trauma. Thus, the clinical hallmark of DAI is the immediate loss of consciousness. Despite the widespread effects of DAI, not every brain cell gets damaged. Usually, in any given area of the brain where a cell is destroyed by DAI, the ones surrounding it survive. Typically, DAI injuries occur as a result of car accidents.

When DAI causes a person to "black out," or lose consciousness, the brain goes "off line" and cannot acquire new information, just as though someone pulled a plug on an operating computer. This occurs because DAI affects very primitive parts of the brain that are responsible for arousal. As a result, there is immediate loss of memory that will never be recovered. Continuing the computer analogy, nothing can get written to the hard drive, so none of one's work can ever be retrieved. When a person is still alive but is in a deep state of unconsciousness, unable to react or respond to any type of stimulation from his external environment, this person is said to be in a *coma*.

Diffuse Hypoxemic or Anoxic Injury

The fourth type of injury, *diffuse hypoxemic or anoxic injury (DHAI)*, is the most serious of all. It involves the loss of oxygen to the entire brain. It is usually the result of an event that deprives the entire brain of its life-sustaining oxygen supply. A person who is unfortunate enough to be involved in a major car accident, for example, might suffer massive internal injuries to the abdomen. If the liver, spleen, or bowels are ruptured, the blood loss into the abdomen can preclude blood from returning to the heart, causing a heart attack. Often a less observable injury, such as a fracture of one of the long bones in the leg, can produce a similar effect that is less likely to be immediately diagnosed at the scene of the accident.

Conditions other than trauma to the brain can also result in oxygen-deprivation that is life-threatening. The most common cause of anoxic brain injury is a massive heart attack that leads to a full-blown cardiopulmonary arrest. If CPR (cardiopulmonary resuscitation) is started early enough, the victim may survive, but if the brain was completely deprived of oxygen for as little as three to five minutes, DHAI brain injury results.

Another relatively common cause of DHAI is near-drowning. As the lungs become filled with water, they are unable to oxygenate the blood, producing all of the effects outlined above. However, especially with children, a near-drowning experience that occurs in near-freezing water may permit survival for a much longer period of time. There have been cases where children have been revived without significant injury to their brains for periods of up to fifty minutes. This seems to occur as a result of the protective effects of lowered body temperature (*hypothermia*), which reduces the brain's metabolic needs. This observation has led to a number of studies in which patients with brain injury have undergone medically induced hypothermia in an attempt to reduce the extent of hypoxemic or anoxic brain-related disabilities. Although the jury is still out on using this procedure routinely following TBI, some of the studies, especially with younger people, have looked promising.

STROKE

A specific type of brain injury occurring as a result of focal ischemic or hemorrhagic injury is stroke. Although not medically classified as a true traumatic brain injury, most people experience stroke as such a physically and psychologically traumatic event that the two disorders have become linked in the minds of many Americans. Although stroke is a very significant cause of neurologic disability in the United States, it is actually classified medically as an *acquired brain injury (ABI)*. Officially termed a *cerebral vascular accident (CVA)*, stroke, or "apoplexy," occurs when one or more blood vessels in the brain gets blocked or ruptures.

Depending on the severity of the damage and the location of the blood vessels affected, stroke victims usually suffer from one or more disabilities, including paralysis or weakness on one side of the body, mood swings, swallowing difficulties, language problems, agitation, and impulsiveness. Some 700,000 Americans have strokes every year, and about 40 percent of them, or approximately 275,000 people, die as a result of their stroke. The majority who survive suffer some sort of brain damage. And although 90 percent of the people who have strokes are over fifty-five, people under that age are not immune.

Those younger than fifty are more likely to suffer a stroke from a sudden trauma to the carotid arteries, which are located in the neck and feed the brain with oxygen-rich blood from the heart. The trauma can be almost incidental, such as a whiplash accident or a chiropractic twist to the neck, events that one would not expect to result in brain injury.

Symptoms of a stroke include:

- Numbness or weakness on one side of the body
- Sudden speech and language difficulties
- Sudden onset of a very severe headache, sometimes accompanied by dizziness
- Loss of vision in one or both eyes, or severe "double vision"
- Confusion in thinking or loss of orientation
- Loss of balance and/or inability to walk, often associated with severe dizziness with nausea and uncontrollable vomiting

Anyone who experiences any of these symptoms should be evaluated at a hospital as soon as possible. Under certain circumstances, early intervention with a medication known as tPA (or tissue plasminogen activator) can dissolve dangerous blood clots 80 percent of the time. When administered within three hours after the incident, tPA, sometimes called a "clot buster," can actually prevent permanent injury. Unfortunately, only one in five stroke victims gets this medication, as few people know what is happening to them during the short time period in which it would be effective. In addition, doctors must be certain that a stroke is not caused by a ruptured vessel, or *aneurysm*, before using tPA, because using a clot buster under these circumstances may be fatal.

One should always err on the side of caution when it comes to symptoms of stroke. If you suspect that you or a loved one may be experiencing the initial stages of a stroke, it's better to go to the hospital immediately, even if you are not sure, than to wait too long and possibly suffer brain damage as a

HEART-SHOCKING

An automated external defibrillator (AED) is the portable version of the disks or paddles used in emergency rooms across the country (and at least once in every episode of the television show *ER)* to deliver a shock to the heart, thereby restoring normal heart rhythms during a heart attack.

Heart rhythm abnormalities can prevent blood from being properly pumped throughout the body and cause a heart attack. In fact, heart rhythm abnormalities are one of the leading causes of cardiac arrest. A defibrillator literally shocks the heart to stop its irregular rhythm, permitting it to resume synchronized beating and reestablish effective pumping. Unfortunately, for every minute that a normal heartbeat isn't restored during cardiac arrest, a person's survival rate drops by 7 to 10 percent.

AEDs help change the equation in the victim's favor. Because they are small, portable, and lightweight, they can be kept in the drawer of a nightstand, at a police station, or next to a fire extinguisher in a school gym. They are designed for laymen and include recorded voice instructions for using them.

result. If it is a stroke, the earlier you go, the more treatment options you will have, and the better your chances of survival and a healthy recovery.

DEGREES OF SEVERITY

Brain injuries vary in severity and can be categorized as mild, moderate, severe, or catastrophic. There are a number of ways that physicians classify severity, so let's take a brief look at the different possibilities.

Mild Brain Injury

Mild brain injury is the most common type of brain injury in the United States and also the most difficult to accurately diagnose. It is usually the result of a brief period of loss of consciousness or disruption of continuous memory (less than twenty minutes). It has the best prognosis of any brain injury: Many individuals fully recover within three to six months following their injuries.

However, because of the brevity of the changes in mental status, many people do not seek medical attention for their injuries. As such, they do not know that potential postconcussive symptoms may interfere with their ability to function at work or school. The resulting mild damage can produce significant disruption in a person's life and in the normal functioning of his or her family. After these disruptive events occur, the victim may seek help, but by then he or she often does not associate these difficulties with the incident. This causes the patient to further delay taking the steps that are necessary to get the right kind of help, and may unfortunately put the brain-injured person's job and/or family life in jeopardy.

Moderate Brain Injury

A person who has been unconscious or has experienced posttraumatic amnesia for up to twenty-four hours has a moderate brain injury and may be transferred to an inpatient or outpatient rehabilitation program once the medical crisis caused by the accident has passed. Some of the symptoms of moderate brain injury include tremors, lack of coordination, weakness, language difficulties, and problems with memory, perception, planning, and judgment. Although the resulting cognitive, emotional, and behavioral problems vary from person to person, most moderately brain-injured people are not ready to go back to work for at least several months or longer.

Severe Brain Injury

A person who is comatose for more than one day and then wakes up is considered to have a severe brain injury. Rehabilitation is generally required and often needs to continue even after the patient has been dis-

THE OVERNIGHT TRAGEDY

We've all seen stories about football players who've been tackled brutally to the ground, or heard the crash of two helmets meeting each other in midair, where miraculously the player may only be stunned, or briefly knocked out. He gets up and the crowd roars as he heads to the sidelines. He sits one out, but by the next play, he triumphantly raises his arms in the air and goes back into the game, again to the cheers of his adoring fans. A true hero! But during the next play, he suddenly collapses and dies.

What happened? Unbeknownst to him and to everyone who witnessed his initial recovery, he had a barely visible skull fracture that ruptured the underlying artery. Good coaches are aware of this possibility and make sure their players get proper medical attention when injured on the field.

charged from the hospital. In addition to undergoing cognitive, emotional, and behavioral therapies, severely brain-injured persons must relearn how to be independent on the most basic levels. The things that must be relearned through intensive training often include social skills and personal grooming habits. Some people improve enough to go back to work, but most likely in a reduced capacity, and perhaps only after several years of rehabilitation. As such patients cannot always manage to achieve complete independence; some of them may need long-term care in a residential facility specifically dedicated to the care of brain-injured patients.

Catastrophic Brain Injury

A brain-injured person who remains unresponsive to the environment and requires total care for all his daily needs is considered to have suffered a catastrophic injury. Although these individuals usually are able to open and close their eyes and have a return of relatively normalized sleep-wake cycles, they cannot speak, follow commands, or even understand what is being said to them. These individuals are often referred to by health-care professionals as being in a *vegetative state*.The speed and completeness of recovery from brain injury depends a great deal on both the severity of the injury and the type of the injury that was sustained.

The very worst outcomes are generally associated with injuries that deprive the brain of oxygen for any extended period of time. Thus, near-drowning or cardiopulmonary arrest following a heart attack leads to significant problems throughout the entire central nervous system, making compensation by healthy areas far less likely than in other types of injuries.

Somewhat better outcomes can be expected from severe and widespread diffuse axonal injury, such as that seen in shaken baby syndrome and large strokes or aneurysmal bleeds. These types of large-scale injuries, in which various brain areas may be virtually decimated, however, prevent nearby neurons from compensating for the deficits caused by the unrecoverable areas.

Less severe, uncomplicated acceleration-deceleration injuries following motor vehicle accidents or tiny nonhemorrhagic strokes usually have the best outcomes. They tend to leave individuals with fewer deficits, and the deficits that do occur often can be compensated for in time. New learning and neuronal reengineering by nearby viable neurons can take place, providing hope for a return to a relatively normal life.

Despite some of the sobering information presented in this chapter, it is important to remember the majority of all brain injuries are mild and have excellent outcomes with appropriate care. Therefore, there is no need to catastrophize and borrow trouble from a tomorrow that may never come. So, now that we've deciphered some of the technical terms you may have encountered, let's move on to the most common myths surrounding brain injury.

chapter 2

Brain Injury Myths

The truth is rarely pure and never simple.
—Oscar Wilde

Ignorance is not bliss, especially when it comes to traumatic brain injury. On the contrary, the more you know, the more you can understand. The more you understand, the more you can accept. And the more you can accept, the more progress you can make in rehabilitation or in helping your loved one.

To that end, here are the realities behind the six most common brain-injury myths. These mistaken—and potentially dangerous—misconceptions live on despite the inroads into traumatic brain injury that researchers have made.

Myth 1: Brain Injury Can Be Detected Immediately

I have been a practicing neuropsychiatrist for over twenty-five years. At least once a month, I hear this myth from bewildered parents who didn't think anything was wrong with their child, from mild brain-injury patients who don't understand what is going on with their own symptoms, or from a patient's loved ones who are confused and afraid. As we will learn in Chapter 4, many cases of mild traumatic brain injury (MTBI) cannot immediately be detected. The signs of this form of brain injury do not show up on scans, X-rays, or simple diagnostic tests, and its symptoms may not crop up for days, weeks, or even months.

Even with all of our advanced diagnostic tools, we cannot always immediately determine exactly which areas of the brain will ultimately be affected, either in mild injuries or in more severe ones. Damage in the frontal lobe area can have far-reaching consequences, causing neurological and chemical imbalances in other areas of the brain, including the limbic system, the temporal lobes, and the parietal lobes. In other cases, however, the damage can be self-contained, causing only slight, temporary injury to executive functions such as problem solving and organizing.

When someone you love is brain-injured in an accident, a heart attack, a stroke, or combat, it is crucial to pay attention to his or her memory, moods, conversations, and habits for several months down the road. Communicate. If anything seems different or wrong, contact your doctor. Early detection can make all the difference between a downward spiral and healthy recovery.

MYTH 2: ANY IMPROVEMENTS THAT CAN BE MADE IN REHABILITATION WILL OCCUR WITHIN A YEAR

The course of brain injury is difficult to predict and depends on the type (or types) and severity of the injury that caused the damage. Most of the healing occurs naturally as the brain responds to the trauma. Unfortunately, medical science cannot yet speed up the process of recovery or replace the brain cells that may have died during the early days following the injury. Healing takes time, and it can't be rushed. The bleeding must stop, the swelling must subside, and bruises must heal. Disrupted neurons must have time to return to full function. Neurotransmitters and hormones must be given a chance to adapt to the new bodily responses that come from an injured brain.

Treatment must be tailored to the individual patient. Early on, this means preventing other complications that may develop in the brain or other parts of the body as a result of the original trauma.

Doctors used to attempt to tell patients and families what to expect following a brain injury. We were well intentioned, basing our explanations on our experience in treating injuries, usually uncomplicated brain injuries caused by motor vehicle accidents. However, we now know that recovery from brain injury can be very difficult to predict. Several different types of brain injury can occur as a result of the same accident. Moreover, even after the brain has done its best to recover, new learning can help an individual compensate for many disabilities that would otherwise leave him severely handicapped and prevent independence. This new learning is hard won. It usually requires an interdisciplinary rehabilitation team to foster its growth, and it may require months or years to accomplish. It also will need to occur in a number of settings, typically a hospital, a residential care facility, and an outpatient clinic.

Miraculous recoveries do occur from time to time. But the majority of them require a lot of hard work by the family, the rehabilitation team, and, most important of all, the injured person himself.

MYTH 3: SHE'LL BE AS GOOD AS NEW!

While the vast majority of individuals with mild brain injuries will fully recover, this is not the case for those who are severely injured. Although many of these patients will experience improvements over time, there is never any guarantee of complete recovery. The reality for severe brain injury, more often than not, is that one must live with some permanent disabilities. They may be overcome, to some degree, but they are still there. Severe brain injury is a chronic condition. It is crucial that we accept it and create a new life from the ashes of the old.

Researchers refer to "the Lourdes phenomenon," the situation in which families go from doctor to doctor, program to program, spending money, time, and energy in the hope that a miracle will occur, that their loved one will come back and be just the same as before. Although second opinions should always be welcomed by competent physicians and rehabilitation teams, the quest for a fourth or fifth opinion becomes more of a distraction from the needed focus on what can and should be done; meanwhile, valuable time slips away. Constant doctor- or program-shopping only fuels the false hope that something or someone will make it all go away, when that is not possible. It is better to work toward acceptance of what *is*, not what might be, without losing hope for the future.

Some factors do play a role in improvement: a good therapist, a good rehabilitation program, or a positive life experience, such as the start of a new relationship or landing a decent job. But it cannot be stressed enough: Improvement from severe injuries does not necessarily mean full recovery. Furthermore, the improvements that occur early in recovery will not necessarily continue at the same pace later on. I've sat with so many families whose hopes soar when they experience the lifting of a coma or the first spoken words of a family member. They believe these break-throughs are signs that complete recovery is just around the corner, but sadly, that is not often the case. When the hoped-for recovery does not immediately occur, they are often so bitterly disappointed that they begin to lose hope altogether.

Although the clock cannot be turned back to a time before the accident, limitations caused by brain injury can be overcome to some extent with compensatory strategies. The limitation may not go away entirely, but there can be improvement. Hope is vital. The difficult steps to independence must be nurtured in order to be sustained. My philosophy has always been that we all will hope and pray for the ideal outcome, but we all need to plan for the probable needs an individual will have when he returns home. If an unexpected outcome should occur, it is far easier to toss those plans out the window than try to make them at the last minute.

MYTH 4: A BRAIN-INJURED PERSON HAS NO CONTROL OVER HIS BEHAVIOR

It's been my experience that many brain-injured survivors and their families tend to experience the emotional and behavioral difficulties that occur as a result of a brain injury in black-and-white terms. They often view the injured individual as either having complete control over her behavior or none at all. The truth lies somewhere in between the two extremes.

GROWING TOMATOES

Alicia has been severely brain-injured for ten years. Even with intensive rehabilitation, she has not regained the ability to be fully responsive to her environment and to be independent. Many people might think the only place for her would be in a bed at home under constant care or in a large, impersonal institution. Unfortunately, two decades ago, that assumption would most likely have been true.

But health care is changing, and some treatment facilities now emphasize the individual needs that such a person requires. Alicia has been a patient of mine for the past nine years. She lives in our specialty medical facility, which is actually a twenty-bedroom house. It is her home. She has her own private room, where she not only has the consistent care she needs but also a patio outside her door where she grows flowers and tomatoes with help from her rehab team. She may not be able to remember people's names or comprehend complex commands, but she can nurture plants. Although her mind may not understand the concept of nurture, I firmly believe that the serenity I see in her face as she intently watches her tomatoes grow from week to week, and feels the warmth of the sunlight upon her face, is a direct result of this pleasing activity that she is able to engage in despite her limitations.

Her family regularly visits her, and her room resembles the one she had at home before her injury. Her parents and brothers have remained just that, her parents and her brothers, as they have not been forced to become her total rehabilitation team, trying to care for her around the clock to the exclusion of everything else in their lives. She and her family have the dignity and pride that she would never have had in a typical institutional setting in decades past. And it shows, in all of them.

When a patient with severe damage to her brain's most sophisticated structures has an emotional outburst, it is rarely because she chooses to have it. Rather, it is because the parts of the brain that would normally control such outbursts have been damaged. Thus, very often, the reaction truly does "go over the top."

However, a person's brain injury cannot and should not be used as an excuse for unacceptable behavior after the individual regains day-to-day memory. Since outbursts of emotion are not acceptable in public, an individual must learn how to control his or her behavior despite the brain injury.

So it's not black or white. The brain injury may explain why such behavior occurs, but the individual must relearn how to control it in order to function independently at home and in society.

MYTH 5: A PERSON WAKES UP FROM A COMA RARING TO GO

Watching the typical movie or TV show, where the star of the show is rushed to the hospital in a coma after being shot by the bad guy, leaves most people with the impression that one day a person is in a coma with tubes sticking out of every orifice of his body and the next day he awakens and begins helping the crime-scene investigators identify his would-be killer.

If only people did come out of comas ready to take on the world! Unfortunately, it just doesn't work that way. The reality is that a person who wakes up from a coma is at first mute and only able to follow people with her eyes. Next, she will be able to respond appropriately to simple commands, and then, if recovery continues, she will begin to speak, but not coherently. She may be confused, combative, and delirious. She may pull at her intravenous lines and attempt to remove the tube that is supplying her oxygen via a mechanical ventilator. Depending on the type and severity of injury, this stage may last from weeks to months. However, after a period of time, her words will become clearer, and eventually she will be able to remember who came to visit that day. She will understand that her IV line is necessary to give her antibiotics. Recovering from coma is a process of healing, not a sudden, total awakening.

MYTH 6: A BRAIN INJURY LEADS TO ALZHEIMER'S DISEASE OR A BRAIN TUMOR

A brain injury happens because of a sudden catastrophic event—an accident, a stroke or heart attack, or a war wound. Alzheimer's dementia, in contrast, is generally a disease process that occurs in genetically predisposed individuals as they age. A brain injury may lead to bleeding or swelling and changes in memory, but it does not *cause* Alzheimer's.

By the same token, a tumor, whether caused by a genetic predisposition, toxic exposure, or some other factor, takes months or years to grow to a point where it impacts brain function. It doesn't just appear one day and— boom!—change your life in a nanosecond. A brain injury does not *cause* a tumor. The injury may lead to bleeding or swelling, but not growth. Tumors grow slowly from cells; brain injuries occur suddenly. They are two totally different things.

However, a brain injury does make a person more susceptible to certain diseases affecting memory. Just as a broken leg can lead to arthritis later on in life, so, too, a brain injury can lead to related diseases. Studies have shown that people who have had a brain injury are at risk of developing Alzheimer's disease and atherosclerosis at an earlier-than-average age. But these diseases are linked to genetic predispositions, environmental issues that are not well understood, and the accumulation of abnormal proteins in the brain.

Fortunately, to be forewarned is to be forearmed. Brain-injured persons can begin taking medicines and make lifestyle changes that may help prevent these problems from occurring.

The bottom line is: Don't borrow trouble from tomorrow when that tomorrow may never occur. Myths are one thing; reality is another. In the next chapter, we'll look at how brain injuries, which are not always obvious, get diagnosed.

chapter 3

DISCOVERING AND DIAGNOSING BRAIN INJURY

Method is much, technique is much, but inspiration is even more.
—Benjamin Cardozo

No one could understand what was going on with Andrea. A once-outgoing teen who was planning to go to college in the fall, she had become, in the words of her mother, a "monster." She shouted, cursed, threw things, and sometimes refused to eat. Other times, she would just stare off into space, or discuss elaborate paranoid theories about those whom she thought were "out to get her." Unfortunately, her parents often fell into the group that she was convinced had the ability to influence her thoughts and feelings in an attempt to "get rid of her." In addition, she was always complaining about pains in her body, which could occur anywhere from head to toe.

By the time she came to see me, she'd been to four general neurologists, three psychiatrists, six psychologists, and one clinical social worker. She had seen a gastroenterologist on the chance that her abdominal pains were the result of an ulcer, an orthopedist because of pains in her shoulder, and a dermatologist to determine if her skin problems were due to some kind of skin disease. She'd seen neurologists to determine if her behavior was the result of a brain tumor or infection. No one had found anything physically wrong with her. Meanwhile, her condition was worsening and things both at home and at school were getting out of hand.

Eventually, the doctors all attributed Andrea's behavior to a profound loss of connection with the real world, a so-called psychosis. They couldn't find anything physically wrong with her, and she was at the age when psychosis usually manifests itself. They had asked her parents if there was mental illness in the family. No. They'd asked if there had been any particular triggers at school that could have added to "typical teenage angst." Again, no. They'd asked if Andrea had possibly taken hallucinogenic drugs, like Ecstasy or LSD. Again, the answer was no, and urinary drug screens were performed to support this fact. Andrea had basically taken good care of herself. Because of her various allergies, she was afraid of taking any designer drugs; she was afraid of what they might do to her.

That's when Andrea's parents brought her to me. The other doctors said Andrea's problems were in all likelihood separate difficulties, but that her primary diagnosis was a psychotic break, probably schizophrenia. Understandably, the specialist physicians involved wanted to treat each problem separately, which meant that her care would be fragmented among different physicians. Her psychiatrist wanted to begin her treatment with medication management of her mental problems, using an antipsychotic medication, while continuing her individual counseling with a psychologist.

However, her parents wanted one last opinion before they began down the path the psychiatrist had outlined. They hoped that a comprehensive evaluation might at least reassure them that "everything that could be done, had been done." They were also searching for a "medical captain of the ship," someone who would be willing to work with all of the physicians involved in her care and ensure that one form of treatment did not adversely affect another. They'd heard about my work as a neuropsychiatrist, and they wanted to see if, maybe, just maybe, Andrea had a brain-based disorder that might tie together all her symptoms and lead to a more comprehensive treatment plan. We needed to dig deep to try to find a diagnosis that would encompass all of her symptoms and that made sense based on the evidence and on solid medical research.

The symptoms certainly bore a resemblance to late effects of a brain injury, but, as the other specialists had pointed out, there didn't seem to be an easy explanation for their current presentation. Neither Andrea nor her parents could recall an accident that might have produced brain injury, and the prior testing had excluded other brain-based disorders like cancer, encephalitis, stroke, or bleeding from a ruptured aneurysm.

DETECTIVE WORK

The doctors who had treated Andrea had all tried to be thorough. But there was one element they had not explored. After a very detailed review of her daily life over the past year, we discovered that she had experienced a gymnastics-related injury at school about six months earlier that had not been viewed as very serious. In fact, although Andrea had been stunned by her fall from the parallel bars, her bodily complaints had eclipsed any concerns about her brain. Yet, given both her physical and emotional difficulties, it seemed prudent to consider the possibility that she was suffering from a form of *complex partial seizure disorder (CPSD)*, or *complex partial epilepsy*. CPSD does not usually show itself like the more typically seen types of total body seizures. The most common of these, *grand mal* or *generalized tonic clonic seizures*, manifest themselves with loss of consciousness and rigidity associated with synchronized shaking movements of the entire body. We decided to perform a five-day video-monitored *electroencephalogram (EEG)*. This is a study that records the electrical activity of the brain while the patient is monitored by a video camera that records bodily movements. If a seizure is seen on the graph of brain electrical activity, we can view the video to see what was happening to the patient's body at that time.

Once the study was read, it confirmed the very intermittent presence of partial seizures coming from Andrea's left temporal lobe. When an electrical seizure was in progress, Andrea was usually unresponsive, staring off into space with very slight lip movements. Once complex partial epilepsy (probably as a result of her fall) became the leading explanation to account for the majority of her complaints, we began treatment with an antiseizure medication. In time, it became clear that an antipsychotic drug was also necessary to help manage her thought disorder. The latter medication was used only for the first few months of her treatment; it was eventually tapered and discontinued. During the next several months, Andrea slowly improved, and many of her bodily complaints eventually no longer troubled her.

Neurorehabilitation must begin with an accurate diagnosis of the underlying disorder of the brain. Without determining what has happened to the brain, how and why it happened, and where in the brain it happened, it is impossible to understand what may happen to the patient as he or she recovers. Without knowing what to expect, it is impossible to appropriately plan for the needs of a patient and his or her family. Studies show that early intervention is crucial, not only to prevent a brain injury from getting worse or having an unfortunate complication go unrecognized, but also to keep a damaged body from developing abnormal responses to the injury that invariably slow future progress.

In Andrea's case, if the trauma to her brain had not been discovered, she would have been inappropriately labeled and her seizures would have continued, quite possibly causing their generalization to the other side of her brain. And if this had occurred, her seizures would have led to full-blown grand mal epilepsy, with all the risks associated with unexpected loss of consciousness and abnormal, involuntary total-body movements.

Diagnostic Techniques

Today's technology and treatment is light years ahead of applying leeches, but we still have a long way to go before we can say that we have conquered brain injury. Thanks to newer and better diagnostic techniques, the percentage of cases deemed hopeless has diminished.

Here, very briefly, are some of the diagnostic testing methods and technologies used in the evaluation of brain injury.

CT Scanning

Computed (or computerized) *tomography (CT)* scans have advanced our ability to see the visible results of brain injury. CT scans collect X rays that have passed through the body (those not absorbed by tissue) with an electronic detector mounted on a rotating frame rather than on film. The X-ray source and collector rotate around the patient as they emit and absorb X rays. Computers then combine the different readings, or views, of a patient's brain into a coherent picture usable for diagnosis.

During a CT scan, a patient lies inside a white, donut-shaped capsule as a technician takes 3-D pictures of "slices" of her brain. With each camera click, the tissues of the brain are peeled away, revealing problem areas not visible with a traditional X-ray machine. One important use for the CT scan occurs in the emergency room as technicians use it to detect bleeding in the brain.

MRI

Combining imaging, physics, and computer technology, *magnetic resonance imaging (MRI)* is even better than CT scanning at looking at both the external and internal anatomy of the brain. Utilizing radio frequency pulses and magnets to image even small clusters of brain cells, MRI converts the resulting signals into a highly detailed picture of the brain, exposing minute details that, in the years before this test became available, would have gone undetected, especially in deep brain structures. However, these machines are more complicated to use than CT scanners and the test takes much longer to perform. Thus, they are not usually used to view the brain immediately following an accident. MRI data are better used in the days after the acute phases of the injury have subsided, when the immediate medical crisis has passed.

PET and SPECT Scans

These tests provide more than just anatomic information about the brain (that is, pictures of the brain structures). When an injected radioactive tracer flows through the brain and is transported inside of healthy brain cells, a *positron emission tomography (PET)* scan creates a map that can evaluate brain function, not just structure. Because it can show functional damage to the brain, it produces a different kind of data that can supplement the information gathered via the MRI technique. These scans let us know whether injured areas of the brain are continuing to function, rather than just giving us a picture showing whether they have been physically distorted or damaged.

Single photon emission tomography (SPECT) is similar to the PET scan except that it uses a more standard and radioactively stable tracer that provides some evidence of brain dysfunction. It is not as specific as the PET scan in determining underlying brain functioning, but it is more readily available and less expensive than PET scanning.

However, it is important to note that neither PET nor SPECT scanning are currently considered clinical tools in the standard practice of managing brain injury. They remain mostly experimental in nature; therefore, your doctor should not be pressured to perform these studies at this point in time. As with many newer technologies, they are likely to be incorporated into standard practice to answer certain diagnostic questions in the future, but not just yet.

EEG

An *electroencephalogram* is similar to an electrocardiogram (ECG or EKG), except that instead of measuring electrical impulses in the heart, it measures them in the brain via electrodes attached to the scalp. It is very important to remember that an EEG can record brain electrical activity only while the electrodes remain attached to the skull. We've all heard stories of people who, after being told by their doctor that they have "a perfectly normal EKG," drop dead from a heart attack the next day. Likewise, EEG readings show us only what is going on in the brain during the time the EEG is actively running; an EEG can miss rare events, and it certainly will not show future electrical abnormalities that have not yet occurred.

Abnormal sharp waves, seen as episodic electrical peaks and valleys, or spikes on a printout, for example, may suggest an underlying seizure disorder, but usually clinical correlation is required to ensure a reliable diagnosis. In severe brain injury, background slowing is often seen on an EEG, suggesting underlying, diffuse brain dysfunction, but that does not provide a diagnosis of what is exactly wrong. It is also very important to remember that the diagnosis of an early disorder does not mean that it will persist. If it does, the diagnosis of epilepsy may be appropriate.

Evoked Potentials

Like EEGs, tests called *evoked potentials* measure electrical activity in the brain, but they take it one step further. This diagnostic tool involves provoking electrical impulses in the brain by means of visual, auditory, and sensory stimuli (in three different tests) to measure the brain's ability to respond. Once an appropriate stimulus has been provided to an area of the brain, the corresponding electrical response is recorded and evaluated so that the technician can determine whether that area of the brain is functioning as it should be electrically, compared with studies of the same stimulus being applied to the same brain area in uninjured individuals.

Neuropsychological Evaluation

In a neuropsychological evaluation the physician attempts to understand an individual's information processing system, that is, how he processes information from the world around him to make decisions and act on them in daily life. There are two components to the information processing system. The first consists of the five basic cognitive processes: attention, incorporation, retention, synthesis, and execution. The second is directed at identifying the efficiency with which the basic processes function. Efficiency factors include speed, endurance, consistency, stress tolerance, and cognitive flexibility as well as psychological variables.

There are a multitude of standardized tests available to assess each aspect of the information processing system. The neuropsychologist selects those tests best suited to assessing the individual's abilities in each area. Issues considered in test selection include the individual's medical status, motor functioning, ability to communicate, and cultural background in an effort to eliminate confounding variables that may interfere with accurate assessment of the patient's ability to process information. Popular and long-standing neuropsychological assessment tools include the series of Wechsler Memory and Intelligence Scales, the Halstead-Reitan Neuropsychological Battery, the Boston Diagnostic and Aphasia Screening Test, the Wisconsin Card Sorting Test, and the Peabody Individual Achievement Tests.

It should be noted that although neuropsychological testing strives to provide accurate, reasonable, and understandable answers to the questions posed by the ordering physician regarding the function of an individual's brain, it is not truly an *objective* test like a CT scan. A CT scan gives results that cannot be consciously altered by the tester or by the individual being tested and is therefore, by definition, an objective test. The answers obtained during neuropsychological testing, in contrast, can be influenced by the patient's level of cooperation with the testing. Thus, it is considered *subjective*. For example, if a person just doesn't want to do the math section of one of the tests, she will score poorly in that area, but that does not necessarily mean that she has a brain injury affecting the areas of the brain most involved in performing basic math.

Often, certain tests developed to evaluate an individual's personality are performed along with neuropsychological testing, and these may also look at specific psychological risks such as depression or thought disorder. The most commonly used personality assessment tool is the *Minnesota Multiphasic Personality Inventory, Revised (MMPI-R)*, which contains validity scales that help determine whether the results are likely to be a true representation of an individual's underlying personality or may be biased by purposeful exaggeration.

I find neuropsychological testing to be most helpful later in the rehabilitation process when a motivated patient wants to know whether she can successfully return to work or school. By understanding her residual strengths and remaining weaknesses, the patient is in a better position to set realistic goals. Often patients can learn to compensate for their weaknesses, with reasonable accommodations permitted by schools or employers. But the information gleaned from this kind of evaluation also

What TBI Is *Not*

Certain conditions may mimic some of the signs and symptoms seen in TBI. But some solid detective work—including blood tests, family history, psychosocial testing, and neurological examinations—can unmask these look-alikes for what they really are. Some of the conditions that should be considered when a person presents with signs and symptoms like those seen in TBI include:

- Chronic fatigue syndrome
- Multiple sclerosis
- Lyme disease
- Clinical depression
- Acute bipolar disorder
- Borderline personality disorder and other disorders involving poor impulse control
- Attention deficit hyperactivity disorder (ADHD)
- Posttraumatic stress disorder (PTSD)
- Brain tumors and other cancers
- Lupus
- Environmental sensitivities and chemical or food allergies
- Sleep disorders
- Macular degeneration
- Migraine headaches
- Rheumatoid arthritis
- Substance abuse

prevents patients from experiencing the disappointment and failure that can come from setting unrealistic goals, or trying to do too much too soon. Obviously, a person who can no longer speak intelligibly would not be expected to return to work as a telephone receptionist, but sometimes the mismatch between abilities and goals is not so clear-cut. One of my

biggest concerns for every patient is to prevent failure and the demoraliza-
tion that accompanies it. A good brain-injury specialist of any medical dis-
cipline should study the patient's family history very carefully, go over his
or her symptoms in detail (especially in cases of mild traumatic brain injury), and look at psychosocial stressors that may complicate the problem.
Such stressors might be tension at home, pressure at work or school, problems in a relationship, or the emotional stress of menopause. Technology
and test evaluations are vital tools in diagnosing brain injury but cannot
completely replace experience, expertise, and good judgment.

chapter 4

RECOGNIZING MILD TRAUMATIC BRAIN INJURY

> *I never knew what hit me and I never realized that after my broken body was healed, my mind would be the final straw that brought the world to an end.*
>
> —Bob Gillen, survivor of an MTBI

The vast majority, some 70 to 80 percent, of all TBIs that occur in the United States are classified as mild. The good news is that many patients with mild traumatic brain injuries (MTBIs), especially the younger ones, fully recover and are indistinguishable from their peers.

The formal definition of MTBI has remained controversial for many years. However, experts from the Centers for Disease Control and Prevention's MTBI Working Group now define it as an injury to the brain arising from blunt trauma or acceleration or deceleration forces with one or more of the following conditions attributable to the brain injury:

- Transient confusion, disorientation, or impaired consciousness
- Dysfunction of memory around the time of the injury
- Loss of consciousness lasting less than thirty minutes or a score of 13–15 on the Glasgow Coma Scale (GCS).

The GCS was developed by a group of neurosurgeons in the mid-1970s who were studying the severity of TBIs in Glasgow, Scotland. They were searching for a simple scale that could be reliably utilized in a test performed in a uniform manner by medical professionals around the world. The factors that emerged as most important in determining the initial severity of TBI involved the patient's ability to open his or her eyes and to perform verbal and motor responses (see Figure 4-1).

Other clinical signs or symptoms may include:

- Seizures immediately following the injury
- Irritability, lethargy, or vomiting following the injury, especially among infants and very young children
- Headache, dizziness, irritability, fatigue, or poor concentration, especially among older children and adults

In another definition, the American Congress of Rehabilitation Medicine says that mild TBI includes only those injuries in which loss of consciousness lasts thirty minutes or less, in which the GCS score thirty minutes following the injury is 13–15, and in which the duration of difficulty for forming new memories—that is, the amount of time that *posttraumatic amnesia (PTA)* persists—is no longer than twenty-four hours. Although these criteria are not without criticism, at present they constitute the most widely accepted definition of mild TBI.

The term *postconcussive syndrome* describes the development of a set of physical, cognitive, and emotional/behavioral symptoms in the days or weeks following a mild traumatic injury to the brain. It is very unlikely that any individual will have every possible symptom following an MTBI. Some will find that their problems cluster around physical issues, such as headaches and blurred vision, while others will mostly experience the symptoms involving thinking (cognitive issues) that can hinder their ability to return to school or work. Still others may find that their worst disabilities are related to the loss of the ability to control their emotions.

The Causes of MTBI

When there is a loss of consciousness for a period of at least several minutes, MTBI is generally the result of *diffuse axonal injury*. In its milder forms,

GLASGOW COMA SCALE

	POINTS TO SCORE FOR TOTAL
EYE OPENING	
Spontaneous	4
To Speech	3
To Pain	2
None at all	1
BEST VERBAL RESPONSE	
Person is fully oriented to self, place & time	5
Confused but understandable conversation	4
Says inappropriate, but understandable words	3
Incomprehensible words	2
Incomprehensible sounds	
None, even to pain	1
BEST MOTOR RESPONSE	
Appropriately obeys commands to move	6
Localizes movement to painful stimulation	5
Withdraws from painful stimulation	4
Abnormal posturing: arms flexed at elbows, feet extended	3
Abnormal posturing: arms extended, feet extended	
None	1

SEVERITY OF INJURY BASED ON TOTAL SCORE
Severe: less than or equal to 8
Moderate: 9–12
Minor: greater than or equal to 13–15

Figure 4-1

DAI does not invariably result in the death of nerve cells in the brain but instead causes a passing disruption in the brain's ability to function by preventing the passage of electrical impulses and the release of neurotransmitters. However, in most cases, actual cell death does occur as a result of the trauma. The damage is microscopic and can be seen only in autopsy studies in patients who die of other causes following a mild brain injury. Although it used to be thought that DAI affected every area of the brain, recent research has shown that the damage tends to cluster in the frontal and temporal areas of the brain. This helps to explain why the most significant residual symptoms of MTBI are in higher brain functions such as focusing the attention and maintaining emotional control.

The important thing is that not every cell in the injured part of the brain is killed or damaged. Since neighboring neurons can extend their connections

LEARNING FROM FOOTBALL PLAYERS

Football players get mild concussions all the time, and researchers have made use of this unfortunate fact in order to learn about the effects of mild brain injuries. In one type of study, all members of a football team are evaluated in terms of cognitive and emotional functioning before the season begins, and then players who experience MTBI are retested later as the season progresses. The initial tests serve as a baseline for later comparison so that researchers can evaluate the effects of any injuries that occur.

Because of the nature of the game, it is inevitable that some players will suffer MTBIs as the season progresses. This subgroup is examined using the same set of tests used before the season began, often for up to a year following their injuries. Although there are always early, measurable deficits—especially in the ability to pay attention—the good news is that, after three to six months, these deficits seem to disappear, or at least are no longer detectable.

There are now guidelines on how many MTBIs a high school football player can sustain before he should be permanently benched. If you are a parent, you can check with your school district to determine what, if any, standards have been set to help protect your young athlete.

to downstream cells, the impairments in MTBI are generally limited to those seen immediately following the injury. However, recovery is still a very slow process, because it requires that remaining healthy cells actually sprout new connections to rewire the links that were affected by the damage.

A Case Study

The experience of one of my MTBI patients, a sixteen-year-old named Alexis, so closely resembles that of the majority of patients that it is worth describing in some detail as a real-life example of what these individuals and their families experience.

Alexis was a lovely aspiring actress who had the good fortune to be playing the lead role of Maria in her high school production of *West Side Story*. One day, during a rehearsal, she twisted her ankle and fell from the stage, hitting her head on the hard wooden floor of the auditorium. She was out cold for several scary minutes. When she woke up, she blinked but was unable to say anything that made any sense. When she tried to sit up, she felt faint and had to lie back down. She could wiggle her arms and legs, and she felt the throbbing sensation in her ankle. In addition, her head began to pound, just like the worst migraine she had ever had. She felt extremely tired, but whenever she started to drift off, someone would wake her up. Those around her knew enough about head injuries to know that she should not be allowed to go to sleep, because if she did no one would realize if she fell into a coma.

Her parents arrived and called her pediatrician, who advised them to immediately take Alexis to the hospital. By the time she got to the emergency room, her headache and dizziness were so bad that she began throwing up. A doctor examined her pupils and asked Alexis to do a number of things that she felt too sick to try. The next stop was the CT scanner, a device that is like a large X-ray machine that permits doctors to visualize the structure of the brain beneath the skull and determine if any abnormalities exist as a result of an accident, such as bleeding.

Alexis was fortunate. The CT scan did not find evidence of bleeding in her brain, and the routine X ray of her ankle revealed no broken bones. She remained at the hospital for another four hours under observation and was then allowed to go home. She was given a shot for her migraine and some pain pills for her ankle. Her family was given the following list of signs to look for to help them recognize complications that might mean Alexis should return to the ER:

- Worsening headache
- Continuing dizziness
- Insomnia
- Extreme fatigue
- Uneven gait, episodes of imbalance or falling
- Nausea and vomiting
- Blurred vision
- Urinary incontinence
- Seizures

Luckily, Alexis showed none of these worrisome symptoms and slept well that night. As instructed by the ER doctor, her parents took her to see the pediatrician the next afternoon. He gave her a once-over and everything seemed fine. Her headache was better, but she was still having some dizziness and trouble with attention and concentration.

She went to school the following day but came home early, as she felt too tired to finish her afternoon classes. She did not feel up to attending rehearsals for an entire week after the accident. Her understudy worked diligently, but Alexis was committed to returning to her role as Maria for the performances. By the time opening night rolled around four weeks later, she was able to perform her role in *West Side Story* (and got a standing ovation!).

By summer, Alexis was feeling fine in most areas of her life. However, she showed signs of troublesome emotional instability, and her pediatrician referred her to me for an outpatient consultation.

CUSTOMIZED TREATMENT

When Alexis and I first met, about three months after her fall, her symptoms included chronic migraine headaches, fatigue, severe moodiness, and uncontrollable irritability. I had her parents attend the first consultation: In matters affecting the brain and its ultimate functional expression through thought, feelings, and self-awareness, it is vital to have both the patient, who can tell me how she feels, and members of the patient's family—in this case, Alexis's parents—who can tell me what they observe. These are two very different pieces of the puzzle, and both are necessary to a full evaluation. I reminded Alexis and her parents that their individual perceptions may be different, but nobody is "wrong."

Alexis's parents were mainly concerned that her grades had fallen during the final semester of the school year and that she was moody and irritable. Alexis, on the other hand, struggled with people being upset with her, and particularly with her feeling that her parents just couldn't understand how her headaches made it impossible for her to continually focus on her schoolwork.

I obtained the medical records from the accident, school reports on Alexis, and Alexis's medical records from before and after the accident from her pediatrician. In subsequent sessions, it became clear that no one had prepared Alexis about what to expect after her injury, and so she thought she was "just going crazy" when she continued to experience memory difficulties, anger, and depression after several months. She didn't understand the connection between these lingering problems and her brain injury. After establishing a therapeutic relationship, I worked with her on a series of goals—related to both the physical and emotional aspects of her injury—that we wanted to achieve:

1. Stop the headaches.
2. Understand what is going on now and learn what to expect in the near future.
3. Figure out why she can't control her emotions of anger and depression.

Tackling the headaches was the most straightforward of the three tasks. I elected to change her medication with the aim of first reducing both the frequency and the severity of the headaches and then ultimately stopping them from occurring altogether. I substituted a new class of medications for the pain and antinausea drugs that she had been taking. Within six weeks, the headaches were gone and Alexis said her moods were more stable. A number of these medications will be reviewed in Chapter 11.

Alexis and I regularly discussed the fact that many of the things that made her feel as if she was going crazy were related to the cognitive effects of the brain injury. We worked on developing a number of strategies that helped her organize her world and bring back the inner peace that came with predictability. Finally, we spent a great of deal of time understanding how her symptoms had reduced her self-confidence and caused her to become more isolated and even depressed. We worked through a course of cognitive-behavioral therapy (CBT), a form of therapy that has been particularly helpful in treating depressed patients, brain-injured or not. In addition, I prescribed a newer-generation antidepressant medication that helped to raise her spirits and reduced the biological symptoms of depression.

INFORMATION OVERLOAD

In this day and age, we are all exposed to an overabundance of "information," especially on the Internet, much of which is inaccurate and misleading. A little knowledge is a dangerous thing, as the saying goes, but inaccurate information can be even more dangerous. Keep this in mind as you are bombarded with information from friends, family members, and even your primary care physician.

Most primary care physicians cannot keep up with all of the latest knowledge in a field as specialized as brain injury. Their medical knowledge has to be a mile wide to deal with the myriad issues that confront them at the office every day. A specialist, in contrast, gains knowledge in an area that is only about a foot long but must be a mile deep. Being buried in the field and working with brain-injured patients day in and day out is the only way to gain true wisdom about how to guide people through a maze that no one ever really wants to know about, let alone experience.

Finally, I reassured Alexis and her parents that the majority of these difficulties would get better with time. Moving on with her life would allow her to have experiences that would restore her sense of happiness. Happiness is something no doctor can order up: It comes from doing things in your life that produce a sense of well-being.

Her recovery wasn't easy and it wasn't quick, but this multipronged treatment approach is one of the few ways of dealing with MTBI that has reliably been shown to help patients. Not everyone with a mild brain injury requires the intensive treatment that Alexis needed, but all MTBI patients need to understand the consequences of their injury for their lives in the immediate future as well as the fact that they will get better with time. Given the variability of the signs and symptoms occurring with MTBI, it would be impossible to outline how such an approach would apply to all cases. The point I wish to emphasize is that there is no "one size fits all" treatment program for MTBI. Each patient must be extensively evaluated by a specialist who can design individualized treatment structured around his or her individual needs.

There are different rates of recovery for the various symptoms that are possible with MTBI. Some may vanish rather early on, while others may linger. This is why it can be so difficult to diagnose MTBI if several weeks or months have passed following an injury before the patient seeks help. The bottom line is that MTBI is a very individual experience and must be treated as such. But the most important thing to remember is that most people fully recover.

PART 2

The Various Effects of Traumatic Brain Injury

chapter 5

How TBI Can Affect the Body

> *I think a hero is an ordinary individual who finds strength to persevere and endure in spite of overwhelming obstacles.*
>
> —Christopher Reeve

Mechanical engineer Chris Barron was nicknamed "Hurricane Brain" by his college classmates because his mind was always going a mile a minute and he talked just as fast as he thought. In April 1987, he was riding on a boat when its captain brought the craft in way too fast, under the branches of a tree growing near the shore. The captain had forgotten that Chris was six-foot-six. One of the low-hanging branches struck Chris in the head, nearly scalping him and rendering him immediately unconscious. The force of the impact knocked him out of the boat. He was in a coma for four weeks.

When Chris woke up, he had some memory problems and cognitive confusion, which is common for people coming back from a coma. He initially thought he was in a hotel room and spotted a strange lady standing in the doorway. He wondered who she was. She was his mother.

But memory loss wasn't Chris's biggest hurdle after his TBI. In fact, he progressed so fast in the cognitive arena that after eight months of rehabilitation, he was offering to rewrite the programs at his facility; his therapists finally gave up testing him. Chris far surpassed what he needed to know to function in society. His mind moved so fast that "Hurricane Brain" once again became his moniker. He spoke so rapidly that he rivaled the best disc jockeys on the radio and was constantly told to slow down.

Chris's main problem was his body. Because his TBI affected the right side of his brain, his left side was numb. (Each side of the brain generally affects its opposite counterpart.) He had difficulty with balance and couldn't walk. His physical constraints made him irritable and moody. His physical deficits created some cognitive deficits as well. Chris had problems with perception, specifically left-side neglect; he didn't realize that there was a left side of the room, a left side of the table, or a left side of the piece of paper in front of him. He'd start writing from the middle of the page and proceed to the right, and return to the middle for the start of every line. He also had difficulty with his fine-motor skills on the left side—for example, with moving his left hand and its fingers, or the toes on his left foot—but since he was right-handed, this didn't seem to matter very much to him or to his family.

Chris was determined to heal. He did his physical therapy exercises religiously. He rolled a ball up and down his left leg, as the therapist had instructed. He practiced using his left hand to do tasks he could do more easily with his right. As his physical symptoms receded, so did his perceptual deficit.

Chris's wife, Karen, told me a story a few months after the accident that showed how determined he was: "Chris was always an athlete and he had been a great tennis player," she said. "One time, while he was still an outpatient, his mom, dad, and sister came up to visit. They decided to play a game of tennis; Chris insisted on joining them. By this time, he was able to walk and his left side was coming back. But there was no way he could play a good game. He was angry at himself and spent the next two days thinking about tennis, the muscles it used, the movements; he practiced on the court. And wouldn't you know it, three days later, he got on that tennis court with his family and played just fine!"

Chris's irritability and mood swings eased as his physical abilities came back. His mood disorder responded very well to Depakote, a medication used to prevent seizures that is also a mood-stabilizing agent; in addition, it can help to prevent migraine headaches. On this medication, "Hurricane Brain" slowed to a tropical storm, and his relationships with coworkers dramatically improved. He was easier to redirect when he became frustrated, and his episodic explosions came under control. He and Karen had a baby in 1989 who has never once seen her father in a wheelchair.

Today, Chris still has some problems with his shortened attention span, although it, too, has improved. He may need directions to get to the newest shopping center in town, but that may be because he's not home very much. He is now an international manager at the same company where he worked as an engineer, and he spends a good portion of the year in Kuwait.

Chris commented to me, "Wish you could give me a golf pill so I could play a decent game."

After a brain injury, a number of medical complications may develop. Each problem needs an immediate and accurate diagnosis and constant medical surveillance; in some cases, surgery may be necessary to prevent long-term problems. These complications include pneumonia, hypopituitarism, autonomic "storms," seizures, sensory loss, loss of motor control and coordination, posturing, spasticity, increased muscular tone, incontinence, headaches, fatigue, and decreased tolerance for drugs and alcohol. Let's look at each one.

PNEUMONIA

Brain-injured people who land in the hospital are subject to the same risks as everyone else who ends up there. When their injuries make them unable to breathe on their own for a period of time, they will need to be intubated and placed on a mechanical ventilator. When air is forced into the lungs by a ventilator to get oxygen to the blood, the body's natural ability to clear secretions is compromised, and sometimes these fluids get stuck deep in the lungs, providing fertile ground for bacteria to grow. This situation often leads to bacterial pneumonia. A person who is in a weakened state immediately following an injury is not as capable of fighting off infections as he was before the injury, and the bacteria often end up infiltrating the bloodstream from the lungs. This condition is called sepsis, and it can lead to an overwhelming infection that the body has trouble fighting even with the newest antibiotics.

Anytime a person spikes a fever, the doctor must immediately check for a source of infection. This means performing a blood count, taking a chest

COMING BACK

One minute she's asleep, unconscious, in a coma. The next her eyes are open; she's looking around. She's awake and completely back to normal.

This scenario, played out over and over again on TV and in the movies, unfortunately doesn't happen in real life. When a person awakes from a coma, it's only the beginning of many stages that occur along the path to full recovery. In reality, the patient may come back for a minute and then go back into the coma-like state. Initially, she won't be able to talk, even if she is not on a ventilator, although she may be able to follow you with her eyes as you move around her room, tracking you while you continue to talk to her.

Next, if things are progressing in the usual stages following a brain injury caused by a car wreck, the patient will be able to follow simple commands, like "squeeze my hand." The next stage of recovery, as she begins to respond to the environment, however, can be one of the most disturbing to many families. From the silence of mutism emerges the agitation, yelling, and moaning that accompany the confused state that a patient is in as she literally reenters a world that she has no capacity to understand. Imagine awakening underwater in a diver's suit, struggling to orient yourself while only remembering having gone to bed at home the night before. This is what it is like for the brain-injured patient who wakes up in a hospital bed, whose memories may be severely affected. It's no wonder that she will be frightened and agitated; she will scream and may cry hysterically. She will probably have to be restrained so she won't hurt herself or pull out life-sustaining lines and tubes.

Coming back from a coma isn't pretty, but it is a sign of hope. Like everything else in life, it just isn't that simple.

X ray, and collecting blood, sputum, and urine to send to a lab for culturing. Usually, when an elevated white-blood-cell count is discovered, a doctor starts a course of antibiotics aimed at a variety of germs. Once the cultures are returned from the lab, showing exactly what type of bacterium is causing the infection, the medication may be adjusted to target that germ specifically. The goal is to prevent the infection from leading to sepsis as quickly and efficiently as possible.

AUTONOMIC STORMS: UNPREDICTABLE FLIGHT-OR-FIGHT RESPONSES

Sometimes an injury to the midbrain and hypothalamus can affect the body's responses to internal or external stressors, causing them to panic at even the smallest of provocations. Changing the position of the injured person can cause the body to respond with an abnormal release of neurotransmitters, such as adrenaline. The patient's blood pressure will shoot sky high; his heart rate will greatly increase, sometimes up to 160 beats per minute; and hyperventilation ensues. As if this were not enough, the regulation of body temperature may suffer. Body temperature, usually a steady 98.6° F, may increase to life-threatening levels of 104°F or more in these situations.

When this happens, medications designed to block the effects of these excessive neurotransmitters must be given, as well as a pain-relieving medication such as morphine. In addition, a cooling blanket is used to chill the body in order to prevent lasting brain damage until the fever passes.

SEIZURES

Major motor epilepsy, or *grand mal* seizures, complete with full-blown convulsions, loss of consciousness, loss of bladder and bowel control, and writhing on the ground, is relatively rare following uncomplicated closed brain injury. However, the risk of the occurrence of seizures increases with bleeding into the brain and with injuries involving depressed skull fractures. Reading about this type of seizure can never truly prepare you for the real thing. These are frightening episodes to watch, especially because they occur so unexpectedly, leaving the uninitiated feeling totally unprepared to respond to what can be a life-threatening event. Some simple guidelines may help you keep a clearer head if they do occur to someone you love.

- To keep the victim from harming himself, hold him on his side, protecting his head by keeping it in your lap or putting a pillow under it.

- Call for help, especially if this is the first seizure your loved one has had. It is essential to call 911 and get immediate medical attention.

- *Never, ever put anything in the mouth of someone who is in the midst of a seizure.* You may have heard that it is a good idea to insert a finger or some kind of stick or tongue-depressor into the flailing person's mouth, so that he will not swallow his tongue. Nothing could be further from the truth—or more dangerous to you or to the person having the seizure. You could lose a finger, and he could end up aspirating vomit into his lungs. Obviously, these are not good outcomes.

- Realize that many seizures will end just minutes after they begin. It may feel like a lifetime, but most seizures last only a few minutes and then stop. The ambulance may even arrive after the seizure has ended. However, a full hospital evaluation is needed to understand the cause of the first seizure. The real risk is that a second may begin just as soon as the first ends. Continuous seizure activity (called *status epilepticus)* can deprive the brain of oxygen, becoming life-threatening.

Depending on the area of the brain that is damaged, the seizure may be more subtle than a major motor seizure. *Partial or focal complex seizures* may cause a patient to enter a dreamlike state without losing consciousness. A sign of this condition is staring off into space and becoming unresponsive to questions or "spacey." The patient may make repetitive gulp-like mouth movements over and over or say a series of nonsensical "words." On occasion, a person having this type of seizure may report that he smells horrible or has episodic abdominal pain. Because this type of seizure disorder does not produce unconsciousness or express its electrical abnormalities with global bodily movements, and can present with a multitude of different and unusual symptoms, diagnosing it is often confusing and difficult.

Although anticonvulsant medications may stop these seizures, like all medications they have side effects. Thus, as is the case with any medical decision, the risks of the seizures continuing to occur must be weighed against the potential side effects related to the medication best suited to treat them. If these are recurring events, the decision to treat them with medications is easier, but many doctors may wait until a second seizure occurs before committing a person to daily anticonvulsant treatment.

About half the people with TBI experience seizures within the first few days following the injury. For the most part, the seizures are temporary: Overall, only 5 percent will still be having seizures later on. The seizures persist, however, in 15 percent of the patients who experience severe brain injuries.

HYPOPITUITARISM: THE RISK YOU NEVER HEARD OF

Often overlooked in diagnostic evaluations, especially because it usually doesn't appear until three months after a TBI, hypopituitarism can result in a variety of symptoms with serious implications.

Hypopituitarism is caused by an underactive pituitary gland and occurs when there has been an injury to the hypothalamus. Without instructions from the hypothalamus, the pituitary gland doesn't produce thyroid-stimulating hormone, growth hormone, or follicle-stimulating hormone—resulting in weight gain, confusion, dry skin, stunted growth (in youths), amenorrhea (absent menstruation), infertility in women, and impotence in men. The good news is that hypopituitarism can usually be diagnosed with readily available blood tests and can then be treated with medications.

SENSORY LOSS

In some cases, depending on the type of injury and its location within the brain, the major disabilities resulting from a brain injury may be sensory in nature. These can occur in senses such as smell and sight or may affect the

way that your brain processes the sensory information you receive from
your skin.

For example, following a motor vehicle accident, the olfactory nerves
(cranial nerve I), which communicate smells directly from the nose to the
brain, may be lost. This happens when the neural connections communicating this information are torn and do not regenerate. Without a sense of
smell, much of what we eat would not taste the same. Our tongues trans-
mit information primarily about sweet or sour, salty or bitter. However,
when these sensations are mingled with the smells of the foods we are eating, we are quite able to distinguish one food type from another and truly
enjoy our food. Without this added sensory component, most things taste
the same and our appetites are diminished.

When it comes to sight, more than our eyes are involved in giving us the
ability to truly see. After some kinds of injuries, especially those caused by
stroke, an individual's eyes may function just fine. But the patient may be
unable to "see" if there is extensive damage to the occipital lobes, the areas
of the brain responsible for translating images from the eyes into an awareness of what the objects are and placing them in the context of the current
environment. The receiving sensory organs, the eyes, remain intact, but the
injured brain is unable to use the information in a meaningful way. In some

---

LOSING CONTROL

Try this simple test. Close your eyes and touch the tip of your nose. Easy,
right? (Unless you've had too much to drink, producing your own chemically
induced brain impairment, which, hopefully, will pass.) But people with
brain damage can have difficulty with this simple movement, and it has nothing to do with how much they imbibe. They can move their arms or legs—
they haven't become paralyzed or lost muscle strength—but they have lost
muscle control. Because the information received from a damaged brain is incomplete, the fine-tuning that is necessary to precisely touch the target cannot
be transmitted to the finger; therefore it wavers back and forth before it
touches the nose.

stroke patients, this condition is called Anton's syndrome. An individual might repeatedly ask, while sitting in a brightly lit room, that the lights be turned up. Or a person may say he does not "see" the couch, or some other object, in the room when asked, but will avoid walking into it when leaving the room. The couch appears to the eye as an impediment to movement, but the brain doesn't understand why.

When other cranial nerves that control eye movement are damaged, the patient may be able to see, and may know what he is seeing, but instead of seeing one object, he sees two. This is often referred to as double vision, but in medical-speak it is called *diplopia*. In this case, the problem has less to do with the brain or the integrity of the eyes than with the muscle imbalance created when the nerves controlling the eyes are not able to work in harmony.

LOSS OF MOTOR CONTROL AND COORDINATION

It starts with damage to any number of brain structures ranging from the neocortex to the brain stem. This leads to communication problems between the nerves connecting the brain to the spinal cord. Depending on the areas that are damaged, motor movement, sensation, and balance and coordination may all be impaired. Various areas, but in particular the precentral gyri of the frontal lobes, control muscle movement on the opposite side of the body from their location in the brain. Therefore, a left-hemisphere injury will affect the ability to control movement on the right side of the body, and vice versa. Disabilities can include the following:

- *Hemiplegia:* Weakness or paralysis on one side of the body, most commonly seen following strokes.
- *Dysarthria:* A loss of oral muscle function that results in the inability to articulate words clearly, even though a patient's knowledge of language is intact.
- *Dysphagia:* An inability to swallow caused by damage to the neurons that control the coordinated movement of the muscles in the back of the throat (*posterior pharynx*) that close the windpipe (*trachea*) while simultaneously pushing a bolus of food into the

esophagus (feeding tube). This condition prevents the brain-injured patient from eating orally, as fluids and foods are likely to end up in the lungs rather than the stomach, which can cause severe pneumonia.

- *Ataxia:* Awkward gait, an inability to coordinate muscle movements, leading to severe imbalance that impairs the patient's ability to safely walk, even though his muscles may be working just fine.

POSTURING, SPASTICITY, AND INCREASED MUSCULAR TONE

Following a catastrophic brain injury, a person may display some rather odd-looking body postures, depending on where the damage has occurred. A *decorticate* posture is typically seen in patients with damage to the *corticospinal tract* (i.e., axonal fibers that travel between the cerebral cortex and the spinal cord). A patient exhibiting decorticate posturing becomes rigid, flexes her arms, clenches her fists, and extends her legs. She will bend her

HARD TO SWALLOW

We give little thought to swallowing and chewing until we lose the ability to do so. It's hard to believe, but the action of actually swallowing or chewing requires many muscles all working in concert. Without these functions, a person may have to have an external feeding tube placed directly into her stomach so that liquid nutrition can be provided, usually using a pump that runs all day and into the night.

A surprise for most families is that liquids are more likely than solid foods to be aspirated and therefore must be avoided. As swallowing improves for the patient, thickened liquids may be safely introduced. But caregivers must be vigilant and never give their loved ones even a sip of water until instructed that it is safe to do so. Because oral feeding is crucial for independence, safely achieving it is of great importance in any rehabilitation program.

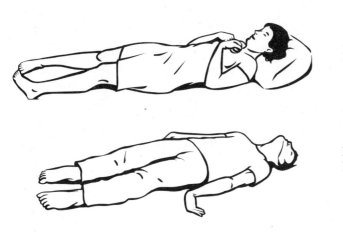

Figure 5-1
Decorticate Posture

Figure 5-2
Decerebrate Posture

arms in toward the body. This posture may get even worse and progress to a *decerebrate* posture. In decerebrate posturing, the arms and legs are rigid, the toes point downward (as the patient is lying down), and the head arches back, all of which indicates the severest of injuries to the brain. Damage to the brain stem is the usual cause of this type of posturing.

Seeing these abnormal postures can be frightening to family members when they first visit a loved one in the intensive care unit. Viewing drawings like the ones presented above may help prepare visitors, particularly children, before their visit. As the immediate medical dangers pass, often a patient will be fit with specialized splints to help control this posturing and permit more flexibility. Intravenous (IV) medications are not very helpful in these conditions, but experimental use of implanted pumps filled with antispasticity medicine has shown promise in reducing the impact of this complication on long-term care. (These pumps are called *intrathecal baclofen pumps*, with *intrathecal* referring to the space between the coverings of the spinal cord and *baclofen* referring to the antispasticity medicine.)

Injuries with lesser severity also present with changes in muscle strength or tone. In some circumstances, spasticity, a disorder of the body's *motor systems*, occurs in TBI patients when certain muscles continually receive an

abnormal message from the brain to tighten. This causes stiffness or tight-
ness of the muscles and may interfere with movement, walking, and, at
times, speech. *The* fingers may curl, the muscles contract, and the patient
may be able to bend her elbows but not release them. Imagine working
with a personal trainer who asks you to do a bicep curl and tells you to
hold the contraction midstream. Spasticity is similar. The one consolation is
that many brain-damaged patients aren't aware that their arms or legs are
frozen.

People with brain injuries can also lose their former ability to be grace-
ful. This has nothing to do with ballet (unless your brain-injured loved one
was a dancer). Dexterity loss is more about coordination, the capability of
muscle groups to come together to jump, run, or skip, or to carry out such
finely tuned motions as playing the piano or knitting. Even holding our
arms out with steadiness requires the contraction and relaxation of many
muscle groups receiving constant fine-tuning from various centers of the
brain. Most often, fine-motor control, like that used in handwriting, is most
significantly affected, as large areas of the brain are devoted to controlling
this activity, just as they are in speaking. When speech is affected, the condition is called *dysarthria*.

Bladder and Bowel Incontinence

It's not pleasant to think about, but muscles in the bowel or bladder—or
their control valves, referred to as *sphincters*—can stop working, or work
only intermittently, when a brain injury occurs, causing incontinence (loss
of control over urinating or having bowel movements). In the case of urinary incontinence, a catheterization (a procedure in which a tube is inserted directly into the bladder) may be performed to permit the free flow
and containment of urine (into a type of plastic bag) as it accumulates in
the bladder. Bowel incontinence is somewhat more messy to manage and
often requires the use of bowel stimulants administered rectally at a set
time each day while a person remains in an adult disposable diaper.

The first focus of neurorehabilitation is to help a recovering individual
regain control of these basic bodily functions by establishing bathroom

schedules that permit the patient many opportunities throughout the day to reestablish reliable control. Unfortunately, a brain-injured person may need to be retaught toilet training from scratch. Obviously, these symptoms need to be addressed quickly, both physically and cognitively. For someone who can't use the bathroom, independence is impossible.

HEADACHES

Studies show that headache pain, on the whole, decreases as the weeks go by following a brain injury. But for someone suffering from postconcussive syndrome or a mild brain injury, headaches can continue, causing great discomfort. Brain injury may trigger migraine headaches associated with dizziness, nausea, vomiting, pain that worsens with bright lights or loud noises, and throbbing pain, often beginning behind one eye. If this type of headache becomes a regular occurrence, medications will be prescribed to prevent them, not just treat their painful symptoms. Great progress has recently been made in both treating and preventing migraine headaches, so anyone who suffers from them should not hesitate to be evaluated.

FATIGUE

A study of fifty-five patients with mild brain injury found that feelings of irritability, fatigue, and anxiety increased *after* the injury as the headaches and dizziness subsided. Brain-injured people need to sleep more than the average person. They need more breaks on the job. They tire more easily after mental or physical activity. Sleep becomes a necessary, sometimes costly, burden.

Alexis's problem with fatigue nearly prevented her from completing school, until we found the right medicine to combat it. This degree of fatigue is worsened when a person faces novel situations that require the use of executive functioning. We all find novel situations fatiguing, and this helps explain why we are usually so tired whenever we travel to a new place: Getting there seems easy, but in fact it requires constant adjustments in our thinking and planning as we cope with situations that we have never experienced before. In the case of a brain-injured individual, this type of adjustment to novelty is required on a daily basis, especially when formal community reentry begins.

During post-acute rehabilitation, breaks for rest or short naps should be planned into a person's daily schedule so that fatigue does not prevent her from fully participating in therapy. Recently, some studies have suggested that a medication generally used to help patients with narcolepsy (a condition where the sufferer tends to fall asleep unexpectedly during the day) may help lessen the impact of fatigue in the lives of those with brain injuries. This relatively new medication, known as Provigil, can substitute for older psychostimulants, which some patients abuse by increasing their doses without a physician's approval as their tolerance to the drug increases.

DECREASED TOLERANCE FOR DRUGS AND ALCOHOL

Imagine that one drink over dinner was enough to make you pass out. Or that a much-desired drink after work made you slide off the barstool. Damage to the brain influences the excitatory or depressing effects of drugs and alcohol. If alcohol makes you depressed, following a brain injury it may make you almost suicidal. And after a brain injury, the brain cells that malfunction from alcohol or drug abuse can ill afford to do so; you need all the functioning brain cells you have!

A word of warning: Many traumatic brain injuries occur *because* of substance abuse, either of drugs, including both prescriptive and street drugs, and alcohol. Such things like drinking while driving, starting a bar fight, or overdosing on a drug can lead to head trauma. Refuse and use wisely, and you'll lower your risk of TBI considerably.

These are, very briefly, some of the physical impairments that can occur after TBI. Family members, friends, and business colleagues can accept someone who, say, comes to work in a wheelchair, needs help cutting his meat at dinner, or needs more than eight hours of sleep. On the other hand, someone who forgets to say "thanks" or acts in irritable and childish ways usually doesn't receive much sympathy.

The fact is that physical problems are easier to adjust to than some of the other sorts of problems that can occur with TBI. Both the victims and their loved ones can adapt. It is the intellectual impairments, the social and psychological inappropriateness, the loss of self that in the long run create the most problems. These are the issues that are the most difficult for patients to recognize and for their families to accept, and they are the most arduous to overcome for successful rehabilitation to take place.

But difficult does not mean impossible. Acceptance and recovery can come with understanding. To that end, let's go on to the cognitive and emotional deficits that can create such havoc and pain.

chapter 6

HOW TBI CAN AFFECT THE MIND

> *The empires of the future are the empires of the mind.*
> —Sir Winston Churchill

Leah Roberts can't remember what happened that September day in 2004. She was at her desk in her office when, out of the blue, she had a horrible headache. "I never experienced anything like it. It was really, really bad," she said. Leah also felt her blood pounding, the pressure going up—way up—and although she was in her mid-fifties, she'd never had problems with hypertension before. A pounding headache, a rise in blood pressure—and that was it. She woke up in the hospital three and a half weeks later, the victim of a stroke. She had problems moving her right side and some right ankle and foot spasticity associated with foot drop that initially made walking impossible. But the worst part? She couldn't speak. She could understand what people were saying around her, but her attempts to speak were mostly blocked, and she could barely force out one or two words. "I could picture the words in my mind, but they just wouldn't come out," she said later, after intensive therapy. "It was frightening!"

Sam O'Connell, of the First Marine Division, Second Battalion Fox Company weapons platoon, in Iraq, was only twenty-four years old when he was the victim of an explosion caused by a suicide bomber outside Fallujah on September 6, 2004. Twelve soldiers died in the blast. Sam suffered massive internal injuries, his face was burned, and his tongue was literally cut in half. He was wearing a helmet, but the explosion shook his brain back and forth inside his head. The force was strong enough to cause a mild traumatic brain injury that left him with a serious postconcussive syndrome.

Although he had several surgeries to repair the physical damage, the syndrome caused by the MTBI was not formally diagnosed until June 2005. Sam couldn't concentrate, follow multiple conversations at the same time, or remember things that had come easily to him before the injury. Nevertheless, he said he planned on getting married and going to college soon.

For teenager Bruce Robertson, it was a car accident. He'd been sleeping in the passenger seat of his friend's car in the Nevada desert when a driver plowed into them. Bruce was literally flung from his seat, flopping around like a rag doll when the car flipped over. Everyone thought that was it; the ER doctors told his family that they should prepare themselves for losing him. His mother, Mary Ann, refused to believe it. For several weeks, Bruce alternated between minimally responsive and confusional states, screaming and flailing his arms when he was conscious, confused and completely disoriented. At one point, Mary Ann literally lay down on top of him on and off for forty-eight hours to keep him quiet and make sure his life-support lines stayed in place. "My son is going to wake up," she prayed. "He will be all right."

Bruce eventually came out of his coma, but he had a severe TBI. He remembers one momentous day at the medical specialty hospital where he was starting the rehabilitation process as he finally emerged from posttraumatic amnesia. The elevator on his floor stood open and seemed to call to him. No one was in the corridor, so he rolled his wheelchair in and got out on the first floor. He headed to the chapel, and slowly, with much effort, got down on his knees and prayed. "Please, God. Bring me back."

The seriousness of Bruce's injury left him with severe posttraumatic amnesia and a prolonged period of retrograde amnesia that prevented him from remembering things that had happened in his life for months preceding his injury. Whether it was his spirit, his youth, his brain healing itself, or a combination of all three, Bruce eventually recovered most of his long-term memory as his retrograde amnesia gradually resolved. He continues to have gaps in his memories of the past, but he has stopped trying to make things up to fill in the gaps and just accepts that he can't remember. When he learns details about his past from others, he writes them in his personal journal so that he can reread them and fit them into the context of his life. He collects associated cues, such as pictures taken during an event, to include in his journal, and these items help to reinforce the memories that he hopes to incorporate. This strategy has served to ease the anxiety he feels regarding his memory problems and has actually provided a way for him to have real data to fill in the gaps that remain.

Today, Bruce's personal journal also helps him to fulfill his new responsibilities as a married man with two children. He is an apartment-complex manager in the apartment complex where he and his family live, and also an ordained minister.

Different ages. Different lifestyles. Different points of view. But one thing the survivors all share is cognitive impairment as a tragic result of traumatic brain injury. Because our learning, memory, intelligence, and problem-solving skills are controlled by the vulnerable structures and connections of the anterior frontal lobes with other areas of the brain, these cognitive deficits are more common than you might think.

What Is Cognition?

The word "cognitive" comes from the Latin verb *cognoscere*, which means "to come to know." Cognition is a very broad topic, and the term itself may be defined differently depending on the context in which it is used. Generally speaking, "cognition" refers to the mental processes by which knowledge is acquired by the brain. These mental processes include perception, reasoning, creativity, and problem-solving skills. Cognition also has to do with thought processes and intellectual functions such as memory and goal setting; it does not include emotional responses.

Cognition requires the ability to *perceive* information. *Perception* involves the use of our special senses (such as sight and hearing) and information transmitted from other parts of our bodies by the peripheral nervous system to inform the intellect about our external environment. Sensory information is translated into organized data that integrate thoughts with external experiences that fully inform us about reality. Damage to the brain following the initial injury can distort an individual's perceptions if the brain's ability to process the information that comes through the sensory receptors is impaired. Such perceptual deficits can affect the higher brain structures that further process this basic perceptional information to integrate thought, judgment, and behavior.

When we engage in the mental activity known as *reasoning,* we use our cognitive abilities to search our knowledge base for relevant information gained in the past that can be used to draw conclusions, solve problems, or guide our social behavior. The most common reasoning strategies include direct retrieval of stored rote information, imaging of similar situations, analyzing the risks or benefits of a proposed course of action, and applying analogies from the past that are associated with our current circumstances. Other strategies involve classifying any new information that is streaming in according to existing categories in our minds and using learned deductive or inductive formal reasoning procedures.

Reasoning by *direct retrieval* involves retrieving a known fact from memory to solve a problem. *Similarity analysis* is typically employed when solving problems in unfamiliar situations. When a solution is not immediately apparent, we typically compare the goal we wish to achieve in our current circumstances with past solutions to problems and select means by which to reduce the differences between the two situations to permit action that can be retrieved from memory. An example might be figuring out how to use a new cell phone's added buttons and features based on one's past experience using the older model.

The restructuring of a problem's presentation that allows prior information of behavioral responses to be used in a novel way is called *insight*. For example, when one uses his knowledge of general carpentry skills and applies it to building something he has never built before, he is demonstrating insight.

Insight is not only used to solve novel problems within the environment; we humans also use it to inform ourselves about our own unique personhood and our behavior. For humans, the highest form of insight is *self-awareness*, that two-edged sword that provides us with historical insight for new learning but reminds us that our lives are finite—a uniquely human understanding that is adaptively "denied" throughout much of our lives. Self-awareness seems to be an activity of executive functioning that occurs in our prefrontal cerebral hemispheres and that relies on the proper functioning of all of our less-sophisticated cognitive functions. A primary cognitive function of all social species is communication. Our species, *Homo sapiens*, is the only one that has developed a communication system based on abstract signs and symbols. Thinking is believed to take the form of a chain of associations among concepts stored in long-term memory, with one thought retrieving others to which it is related, leading to the ability to reason and learn from experience.

The cognitive impairments associated with brain injury are often the weakest links in the chain of recovery that affect a patient's ability to live independently. Without well-functioning cognitive abilities, a person cannot budget for expenses, navigate her way around a supermarket, buy groceries, and prepare healthy meals. She can't easily focus on adding or subtracting, and so has difficulty balancing and maintaining a bank account without bouncing checks. She can't sequence the steps necessary to sort the laundry before it is washed, or recall the social graces necessary to make eating at a restaurant an enjoyable experience.

The worst aspects of cognitive impairment are often related to failures in reasoning and judgment that may lead to the inadvertent injury of the impaired individual or others. These deficits are the reasons that many brain-injury survivors require constant supervision. Furthermore, these deficits impair social functioning that is vital for independent living. For example, the cognitive impairments associated with frontal dysfunction often impact a person's behavior in such a way that he is unable to use abstract thought, which is so important in understanding the behavioral signals that another person exhibits during any social interaction. This lack of awareness often shows itself as an inability to express empathy for the other individual's personal needs, jeopardizing the interactions that are such an important part of maintaining community, family, and intimate relationships.

Because these cognitive impairments affect every aspect of a person's life, they must be understood and treated as best they can. Given the great diversity of people and the nature of their injuries, there are numerous strategies used in neurorehabilitation to help remediate remaining strengths and compensate for deficits.

There are many aspects of cognitive functioning that must ultimately converge to produce new learning and permit one to use good judgment to solve the common problems that we all face in our daily lives. Cognition throughout life can be broadly described as an interaction between knowledge-driven processes and sensory-experiential processes and between consciously controlled processes and unconscious, autonomic processes.

Because the ability to learn is so dependent on the ability to both create and retrieve memories, we will first focus our attention on memory—what it is, how it works in the brain, and how deficits in different types of memory contribute to cognitive impairments that affect reasoning, judgment, and self-awareness, not just the ability to recall events.

MEMORY

Memory is defined as the ability of the mind to store and recall past sensations, thoughts, and knowledge or retrieve this information if it was previously known. It is commonly thought of as the sum of everything retained by the mind. A number of different brain areas are responsible for performing the necessary cognitive functions that permit memories to be made by attending to salient aspects of our experiences and manipulating these data in real time to actively solve problems as they occur. Then, this information must be stored within our brains for future use. Finally, we must be able to retrieve these memories when they are needed to guide our thoughts about how to solve novel problems and use judgment in applying this knowledge to circumstances that are not exactly the same as those previously experienced.

There are several types of memory that may be damaged by brain injury and therefore have an impact on cognitive rehabilitation. These are sensory memory, short-term memory, and long-term memory.

Sensory and Short-Term Memory

Sensory memory is a very brief type of memory that permits us to look at an object and remember what it looked like after a very brief period of observation. This type of memory cannot be prolonged by practice and therefore is rarely able to be regained after brain injury.

Short-term memory, often thought of as "working" memory, provides a relatively short time for people to keep something in mind after it is first learned or experienced (but certainly much longer than sensory memory), thereby permitting the brain time to decide if the information is (a) important enough to be transferred to storage in long-term memory, or (b) unimportant enough to be dismissed as irrelevant and purged from one's thoughts. Short-term memory is very dependent on the ability to pay attention, remain calm, and concentrate on information before it passes into history. It is therefore impossible to accurately predict the exact amount of time that information in short-term memory will be available to any given individual.

Cognitive rehabilitation helps patients retain information by writing it down before it is forgotten. Patients are encouraged, for example, to write down information from telephone calls before they forget they occurred. This compensatory strategy permits individuals with impaired short-term memory to transfer information into a longer-term written medium that enables them to recall it at a later time, even if it is not translated into long-term storage.

Long-Term Memory

Long-term memory is a complicated process and has several components that most family members will hear about during the acute recovery stage and neurorehabilitation. There are many different forms of long-term memory. However, the two major subdivisions of long-term memory are *explicit* and *implicit* memory.

Explicit memory is also commonly called *declarative memory*. It requires making a conscious connection between the parts of our brain that permit us to understand the meaning of new information. Language and the associative areas of our brain, including the prefrontal cortex, permit this new information to be stored and put into context according to the time period when something occurred or came to our attention. Explicit memory also ties this information to past memories that are similar to the new learning to help us retain the information in the future. To that end, explicit memory is often associative, in that our brains link similar categories of memories together. As an example, think of the number of associations that most people have when they hear a simple word, such as "car."

Explicit memory can be further divided into *episodic* and *semantic* memory. *Episodic memory* provides us with an ongoing account of what occurs in our lives over time. It records memories according to the time at which they occur in our lives; that is why memories are often associated with specific dates and times. The return of episodic memory marks the end of posttraumatic amnesia following acceleration-deceleration brain injuries. It is episodic memory that permits us to remember what we had for breakfast or who visited us during the day. This form of memory appears to be primarily located in the hippocampus of the brain.

Semantic memory, the other type of explicit memory, can be thought of as "textbook learning," though it does not come only from textbooks: It includes knowledge that we learn from others when they tell us information from their own experiences. Sometimes it is referred to as *crystallized memory* because it is so stable and remains even following severe brain injuries. It is the type of memory that permits us to recall that George Washington was the first president of the United States. Research scientists have not completely localized the parts of the brain that are responsible for this form of memory.

Implicit memory, also called *muscle memory*, is very different from explicit memory in that it doesn't require conscious thought and permits us to perform many daily routines by rote. Implicit memory also embodies what is known as *procedural memory*. It is because of muscle memory that we can carry out common repetitive tasks without consciously thinking about them. Muscle memory enables someone to remember how to ride a bike even after years of inactivity. Other examples are tying our shoes and brushing our teeth. This form of memory also provides the foundation for what we think of as our natural abilities, such as walking, throwing a ball, or lifting heavy objects. Often, the more we consciously think about performing these activities, the less able we are to precisely perform them, because when we use parts of the brain that are usually reserved for novel activities, it tends to disrupt the natural flow of tasks performed using procedural memory, such as dancing.

The important thing to remember about procedural memory is that it uses different parts of the brain than the other forms of memory. This is why even when brain-injury survivors do not retain the ability to use explicit, long-term memory, they can be taught to perform activities of daily living (ADLs) by using implicit memory. However, teaching a person to relearn tasks via implicit memory takes far longer than utilizing explicit "talk" memory, because to translate these activities into rote motor activities requires a great deal of rehearsal and repetition.

Permanent Amnesia

The most profound type of memory difficulty sometimes occurs after prolonged oxygen-deprivation to the brain caused by cardiac arrest or near-drowning. It is a global and often permanent amnesia that results from severe dysfunction of the hippocampus and the anterior frontal lobes. In these situations, although a survivor can attend to what is said and even repeat it back to you, she cannot consolidate the information into long-term storage, a function that is associated with the hippocampus. Ask her what you just said, and she'll have no problem. But ask her five minutes later, and she won't remember. She is able to perform immediate recall, but there are no memories being created, consolidated, or stored.

Retrograde versus Continuous Memory

Another way to classify memory is in terms of *retrograde memory* versus *continuous memory* (also known as *prospective memory*). These terms are commonly used in rehabilitation. Retrograde memory refers to memories of things that happened in the past. If a patient is said to have "retrograde amnesia," that means she has lost her memories of events that occurred prior to the injury.

Continuous, or prospective, memories are the ones that are formed continually, each day, as we live our lives. Those suffering from posttraumatic amnesia after a brain injury are unable to lay down new memories. Thus, a patient may not remember what she had for breakfast that morning or who came to visit her that very afternoon. The return of continuous memory is an important landmark in recovery from acceleration-deceleration brain injuries because it often heralds the end of the need to provide constant supervision for a previously amnesic patient in order to provide for his or her safety.

APHASIA

Other specific brain functions, particularly those involving speech and language, greatly impact our ability as humans to symbolically represent our thoughts and therefore deserve some discussion in this chapter. In TBI, these functions can be severely compromised by aphasia.

Aphasia is defined as the loss of speech and language, and occurs when there is damage to specific areas of the brain that make it appear as though a person has memory problems. However, the true cause of the brain-injured patient's inability to express himself and effectively use memory is related to damage to the areas of the brain responsible for speech in the left precentral gyrus of the frontal lobe, in the postcentral gyrus of the parietal lobe, and in the anterior temporal lobe.

There are many different classification systems for aphasia; however, the one adopted by the National Aphasia Association divides aphasia into two broad categories: fluent and nonfluent.

Individuals with *fluent aphasia* have problems understanding spoken and written language. This type is also known as *sensory aphasia* or *Wernicke's aphasia.* In this case, the injured individual will be able to say both real and nonsensical words, but their sentences have no meaning because they cannot find the nouns, verbs, and adjectives that would accurately express what they are trying to say. Their speech is often described as being like a "circular word salad"; they are saying words and stringing them together into "sentences," but the words they have chosen do not make sense together. In fact, they sometimes make up words that do not exist.

People with *nonfluent aphasia* have difficulty communicating both orally and in writing. This type of aphasia is also called *motor aphasia* or *Broca's aphasia.* These individuals understand language but cannot describe their needs beyond blurting out a few nouns. As this type of aphasia improves, a listener can usually get the idea of what a person with a nonfluent aphasia wants to communicate.

The most severe form of aphasia, *global aphasia,* involves injury to all of these areas of the brain and is often exhibited immediately following an injury. Global aphasia makes it impossible for a person to speak or comprehend language, whether it is written or oral. However, in most cases, global aphasia resolves into fluent or nonfluent aphasia.

There is no way around it. When memory becomes impaired, it will affect learning, which, in its most basic form, is committing new information to memory, integrating this information into our experiences, and using it as a frame of reference in our individual, daily lives.

Without memory, we cannot process and store information.

Without the ability to process and store information, we cannot learn.

Without an ability to learn, we cannot create new memories, or reason, or find novel ways of solving new problems.

Memory loss. An inability to conceptualize or solve problems. A sensory deficit. Lack of insight or imagination. These effects on the mind caused by injury to the brain add to the difficulties that brain-injured people—and their families—will face in adjusting to their new circumstances.

These deficits can also prevent solutions from being found—sabotaging many rehabilitation strategies that rely on these basic functions for successful implementation. How? Impairments in self-awareness or the inability to relearn ADLs using declarative learning severely limit the pace at which new learning can occur, and some patients and families just give up because of the prolonged time frames necessary for successful rehabilitation. It may be because they are discouraged, or it may be because their funding sources simply dry up. But the good news is that there are neurorehabilitation centers that can achieve goals with TBI patients that were once seen as unobtainable. Evidence-based medical strategies have come a long way and can now overcome many things that were obstacles in the past. (The management of TBI-related disorders will be covered in Chapter 12, "Cognitive Therapy.")

But before we look at the treatment and rehabilitation process, it's important that we first understand how TBI may affect your loved one's social behavior and emotional life.

chapter 7

How TBI Can Affect Social Interaction

"Though this be madness,
yet there is method in 't."
—William Shakespeare

Donald Thweatt had always been strong, healthy, and brave. As a young-ster, he was the captain of the softball team: He gave the orders and the other kids listened. He always knew he wanted to become a soldier when he grew up. While still a teenager, he joined the Civil Air Patrol to help with search-and-rescue operations. He joined the National Guard after gradu-ating from high school and was soon a first lieutenant in the U.S. Army Re-serve. As an adult, he weighed about two hundred pounds, all muscle. He went to the gym almost every day and could bench-press close to three hundred pounds. He had a good job as a manager at a computer data com-pany, a wife, and an adorable child. Life was good.

On August 5, 1990, Don was called up to serve in Operation Desert Shield, and was told to report to a base in Pennsylvania. It was there that he became a victim of TBI.

Don now incorrectly believes that his army buddies beat him up because they were jealous. But the more likely story is the one told in an article in the *St. Louis Riverfront Times.* This version, provided by eyewitnesses and army reports, goes something like this: There was a night of drinking at the Pennsylvania Tobyhanna Army Depot. Don was sitting in the center seat of a sliding-door van with the door open. It is not clear how fast the van was moving, but to avoid hitting another car, the driver swerved off the road. Don leaned over toward the door, which hit him on the right temple. He supposedly said, "Damn, that hurt."

He seemed fine. He and his buddies made it back to their barracks with barely a scratch. Before falling asleep, Don complained of a headache. He woke up a few hours later and vomited into a drawer in his bureau. At 5:30 A.M., one of the other soldiers found him lying unconscious in the hall. He was rushed to the hospital.

The diagnosis? An epidural hematoma—bleeding from a ruptured artery that had formed a clot outside the dural membrane of the brain. Emergency surgery was performed. A second brain surgery was also required to release pressure that had been building up. Don's prognosis was grim. The neurosurgeon told his parents that he'd need to be institutionalized for life.

Then, things got worse. Don's parents decided to take care of him instead of putting him in a hospital. At first, Don did nothing more than cry, waking his parents in the middle of the night because he was scared. They bought a hide-a-bed so he could sleep next to them. He gained over two hundred pounds, but his past strength meant that he was still a formidable man.

He developed a violent temper and threw glass soda bottles through the windows of his parents' house; he threatened them. Soon, Don's family members began to fear for their lives. The last straw was when he insisted on driving. His father didn't think it was a good idea and said no. The next thing his dad knew, Don pushed him out of the driver's seat one day and took control of the steering wheel. When his father got out of the car, Don tried to run him over. The police soon showed up. Don's father was standing between two parked cars for protection. "Were you trying to kill him?" the policeman asked Don.

That's when Don's parents knew they couldn't do it alone.

For years, Don was shipped around to various veterans' hospitals, nursing homes, assisted living facilities, and rehabilitation centers. For a time, he even lived in his car. Finally, he landed in jail, convicted of attacking a nurse at one of the facilities. In prison, he attacked a guard. His wife divorced him, and his parents were terrified of him. He had no friends, no allies, not even a doctor he could consistently see and trust.

By the time Don came under my care, he seemed to be a hopeless case. Even his court-assigned legal guardian had never seen anyone like him— and he had over 450 people on his caseload at the time. Today, Don resides at our residential brain-injury rehabilitation program where we are slowly working with him on anger management, patiently and carefully. On occasion, he requires some sedation, but he can now do all of his own activities of daily living, including doing his laundry and making his own lunch.

Out of jail? Yes. Progress? Yes. Independent? No. And although there will only be very slow progress in the future, his ability to maintain this progress for any predictable period of time remains in question.

Don Thweatt's case may be extreme, but it reflects the fact that the psychosocial factors of TBI can have far-reaching implications, creating problems in school, on the job, and at home. We understand why behavior becomes disturbed when the brain is injured, and we even know the behavioral patterns that may erupt. But the way they are displayed is as unique as the person himself—from Don's violent outbursts to another person's interrupting, cursing, or saying things at the wrong time.

OUT OF WHACK

Sometimes, paradoxically, inappropriate behavior is the result of improving self-awareness—a depression or anger that springs up when someone finally realizes she is disabled, that he has lost the last three years of his life, that she can't walk without a cane, that he can't think of a word that's "on the tip of his tongue."

Other behavioral problems stem from deficits in self-awareness and impulse control, which may be caused by damage to the inhibiting areas of the brain. When brain cells are damaged, they lose their ability to maintain the intricate electrical and chemical balance necessary for normal brain function; as a result, disturbances of the brain manifest themselves as disorders of the mind. Consequently, everything gets out of whack. With the inhibiting neurotransmitters "out to lunch" and the excitatory chemicals the "barbarians at the gate," the brain goes haywire, turning into a wild, out-of-control machine, which can translate into the TBI patient saying and doing embarrassing things, acting wild, even becoming violent.

When deficits result in behavioral changes, they create psychosocial dysfunction because it is the brain that creates our unique personalities and exerts control over all of the behavior that we demonstrate to the world. In order to function in society, we must be able to work together with others to get even our basic needs met. And although we all have bad days now and again, brain injury can make each day such a trial for the individual and those around him that it pulls apart the fabric of their social interactions. Isolation can become the rule rather than the exception as a result.

Anger Versus Not Caring at All

If damage occurs in certain parts of the anterior frontal lobes that are ultimately responsible for exercising higher order control over our emotions, the more primitive emotion-generating areas of the brain cannot be held in check by executive functioning. When a patient inappropriately expresses these emotions, he is said to have *episodic dyscontrol syndrome (EDS)*. As in Don Thweatt's case, angry and possibly violent outbursts will occur as a direct result of this dysfunction. These episodes will start up suddenly and may be:

- Explosive but often undirected
- Dramatic
- Unpredictable
- Uncontrollable (in that once they begin they are rarely able to be stopped by the individual himself until they "burn themselves out")
- Brief

Sometimes EDS will not show up for months after the accident, until the individual has completed rehab and gone home—back into the real world. It may be triggered by a stressful situation, even something as trivial as one of the standard annoyances of life, such as traffic, a broken appointment, or a burned dinner.

EDS is not the only possible outcome of damaged frontal lobes. When the damage is more restricted to the outer, side areas of the frontal lobes, known as the dorsal lateral areas, the person may have a very different sort of disorder. Instead of showing anger, she may just not care about anything, showing little motivation and interest in the life going on around her. In these situations, she may be content to sit in front of the TV all day, not even bothering to change channels. With this type of injury, the affected person does not usually initiate spontaneous interaction or behavior—not even the behavior necessary to perform the routine activities of daily life. Often she shrinks into herself, creating a very small package. This type of injury may be confused with depression, as the symptoms are similar, but rather than feeling helpless and hopeless, the individual just doesn't feel at all. She isn't suicidal, because she is unaware that anything is really wrong.

Both expressions of frontal injury are called *frontal lobe syndromes,* and both are dysfunctional, but one is more obvious and potentially dangerous and gets more attention in discussions surrounding brain injury.

The good news is that these brain-injured patients manage to come through their accidents with many of their other cognitive abilities intact. The bad news is that their personalities go through tremendous changes because of the damaged brain structures involved. Neuronal connections that used to relay information to other parts of the brain that were essential to inhibiting emotional outbursts or initiating behavior have been disrupted.

In summary, some psychosocial symptoms of frontal lobe syndrome may include:

- Lack of motivation
- Impaired social judgment
- Increased risk taking
- A lack of regard for future consequences—a "live for today" mentality
- Failure to recognize the effect of one's behavior on others

- Increased libido, but decreased control over when to express it
- Poor grooming and daily hygiene
- Loudness
- Perseveration (repeatedly asking for the same thing over and over again, even though the request has been granted, as if the person is stuck in the same groove of a vinyl record album)
- Indifference to the needs of others

In patients with frontal system deficits, inappropriate behavior can occur *despite* the fact that other basic cognitive abilities are intact. On the other hand, this behavior can also occur with the more global cognitive impairments that can result from severe brain injuries. Self-regulation, including the ability to know right behavior from wrong, to act in a mature manner, and to summon up self-control, is another component of executive functioning—just like goal setting, planning, thinking, and taking initiative.

In other words, psychosocial disturbances can be a direct result of a brain-injured patient's executive dysfunction—or a part of it. Without an ability to think conceptually (taking in visual and language cues from another person and from the environment), there can be no analysis of a given situation (determining the mood of the other person, figuring out the meaning of his actions, and understanding other things occurring in the environment). Without this ability to analyze one's surroundings, there is just the impulse to act, regardless of the consequences.

INAPPROPRIATE AGGRESSIVENESS

Inappropriately expressed aggressive behavior is one of the most disruptive symptoms after TBI, with a real potential for harming both the patient and his loved ones. As we saw with Don, violent behavior associated with TBI can lead to prison. One study found that 82 percent of the prisoners doing time in our jails had had at least one TBI before their incarceration, and 65 percent of these prisoners had lost consciousness more than once as a result of a traumatic head injury. More troubling was the finding that the prisoners who'd experienced prolonged loss of consciousness (usually for a period of more than thirty minutes) had gotten treatment, while those with mild brain injury had not. In other words, the majority of prisoners were suffering from a mild brain injury that had remained unrecognized and untreated.

Some form of aggressive behavior is also common in the first few months of rehabilitation. Studies have found that anywhere from 11 percent to 96 percent of all TBI victims will become at least temporarily violent; while this is quite a large spread, these data demonstrate the difficulty that even trained professionals have in defining exactly what constitutes an act of aggression. For some, cursing alone counts as aggressive; for others, an act is considered aggressive only if someone actually gets physically hurt. The result of this confusion is that studies involving the management of aggressive behavior are not easily generalized so that the information may be used in different patient populations and treatment settings.

Further complicating matters is the context in which aggression occurs. For example, the confusion a patient experiences in the early stages of recovery following a coma universally leads to some expression of what can be interpreted as aggression as an individual attempts to cope with the very alien environment of an intensive care unit. Suddenly, the patient awakes from a very deep sleep, unable to move, unable to speak, often with a tube down his throat, in pain and in a strange, noisy place. Compounding the problem is that many TBI patients also have hallucinations during these early days. Finally, as the confusion recedes, the hallucinations pass, and rehabilitation begins, a general feeling of irritability moves in that can last for a few days or several months.

The good news in all this? Most likely this injury-induced aggressiveness will be gone before the year is out. Unfortunately, the agitation sometimes takes on a life of its own, occasionally lasting for a longer period of time. Then, it can become a habit, a *learned* response to stress that rears its nasty head whenever social, financial, or personal problems pile up.

The anger and frustration peak as disabilities become more and more apparent and as awareness of one's limitations increases. Indeed, reality can be so difficult, so compromised—physically as well as psychologically—that many people with TBI refuse to admit (or are incapable of admitting) their disabilities exist for years after the incident. Refusing to accept your limitations once you become aware of them is one thing. How-ever, there is a brain-based disorder usually associated with compromised frontal function, called *anosognosia,* which involves not just stubborn re-fusal to admit that you have problems, but also a true lack of ability to un-derstand that they even exist.

Another type of deficit in awareness, usually referred to as a *neglect syn-drome,* is seen in patients with large right hemispheric strokes; such a patient can actually be shown his left arm and adamantly deny that it is his. In fact, this lack of awareness causes the patient to neglect to even wash this arm. This form of neglect is also seen in a patient's reaction to objects in her left visual field. This was demonstrated in a classic experiment in which patients instructed to fill in the numbers on a drawing of a clock filled in only one side, pushing all twelve numbers onto the right half of the circular face of the clock. Newer research on neglect shows that nearly 45 percent of severely in-jured patients with this symptom never regain complete awareness of those internal and external aspects of their bodies and their external worlds.

Although statistics are just numbers that reflect a general population, never any given individual, they can be useful in helping doctors predict what patients may experience as they recover from injury. The following risk factors may predispose TBI patients to aggressive behavior:

- Under thirty-five years old
- Poor social function prior to the accident, including aggressive and antisocial behavior and bullying
- A history of alcohol or drug abuse
- The diagnosis of a type of TBI or ABI (acquired brain injury) associated with the behavior, a severe TBI or ABI, or a TBI or ABI affecting a part of the brain associated with the behavior
- Prior psychological or psychiatric problems, including depression, bipolar disorder, or impulse-control personality disorders

Of course, these risk factors are generalizations and may not be relevant in your loved one's case.

Even when someone close to a TBI patient realizes that the anger a loved one is expressing is a result of dysfunctional brain anatomy or the re-sult of becoming aware of a painful reality, the anger still hurts. Period.

Unfortunately, the anger is usually directed at those closest to the brain-injured person: his family, his friends, his therapists, and his rehabilitation team. Even more unfortunately, this anger can quickly turn to physical aggression, like Don's did, which translates into destroyed property or a direct hit to someone else's body. At McLean Hospital in Boston, where I did my residency, all the patients on my unit had only one TV set, and they had to agree on which show to watch. When one patient changed the channel, he was attacked by another patient who apparently didn't agree with the choice of show. So much for enforced collaboration!

At least this aggressive act was committed within the confines of a hospital. What if this same patient had been in a store, growing angrier and angrier at a salesperson because she wasn't checking him out fast enough at the register? The clerk wouldn't know that her customer had a TBI; she'd just see an unruly individual. She would either ignore his finger-tapping and angry expletives or try to explain that she was working as fast as she could. But the patient, worried because he didn't know how to count his money, and anxious that he might give her the wrong amount, could become frustrated and angry. He might become more and more certain that the salesperson was testing him, taunting him. He might strike out at her. The next thing you know, he's in big trouble.

This scenario happens more frequently than you might think. I've had hundreds of patients threaten their spouses or parents. I've had patients who wanted to burn down their houses or destroy public property.

Add to this the extreme emotional ups and downs that TBI patients experience as the result of damage to their limbic system (which is believed to be the biological foundation of our emotions), and you have a person who is out of control, often through no fault of his own.

"Yes, Please" and "No, Thank You"

Manners are learned and so is appropriate social behavior. By the time a reasonably normal person is a teen, social rules, customs, and taboos are usually ingrained and in sync with the rest of the world. However, brain injury can destroy all that we know about saying thank you, using a knife and fork when eating, or zipping up our pants before we go out in public.

Brain-injured people are often not aware that they're acting rudely or lewdly. Throwing the mashed potatoes and gravy across the room in anger or frustration feels just fine, thank you. Ditto for the lamp, the chair—or the nurse. But as difficult as it may be, you must always try to protect yourself and your loved one from the harm that can result from these behaviors. If at all possible, it is best not to take these explosions too personally; remember that they are caused by the brain injury, not mean-spiritedness. Although brain injury is no excuse for disruptive behavior—and the individual must relearn how to control it—nonetheless, it isn't done just out of spite.

Unfortunately, one of the ways these deficits show themselves in TBI patients is in the expression of extremely rude social behavior: calling therapists and nurses terrible names, using religious or racial slurs (especially the "n" word), and sounding like a bigot. Think of it as a manifestation of basic impulses being expressed without screening for social appropriateness, because of disinhibition and the mistaken belief that such conduct will get a person what he wants—just to be left alone. When she doesn't feel like doing therapy, the easiest way for the TBI patient to drive off the therapist, short of hitting him, is to call him every name in the book to get him to go away.

Unfortunately, when therapists take these insults personally, it only reinforces the power of the TBI patient to prevent further rehabilitation. So these issues must be dealt with by mature, well-trained, compassionate therapists who know they are going to get the job done regardless of what comes out of a patient's mouth. An experienced therapist has heard it all before—and more. These types of psychosocial problems can indeed try the patience of a saint, let alone a therapist, but when the therapist understands them as symptoms of the brain injury, the TBI patient can still make progress in the therapy sessions over time.

Sexual Dysfunction

Sexual problems are nearly universal in traumatic brain injury, and they are one of the primary reasons that married TBI patients so often get divorced. Damaged frontal and temporal lobes can affect sex drive by taking away

---

DID YOU KNOW?

- People who have accident-caused TBI are 9 percent more likely to experience manic episodes—with their impulsive, sexually uninhibited characteristics—than people who have had strokes.
- Sexual dysfunction can be caused by some of the medications TBI patients need to take, including antidepressants and antiseizure drugs.
- If birth-control pills have been prescribed to them, many people with TBI need to be monitored because they will forget to take them. They may also forget to use condoms to ensure "safe sex."
- A person with a brain injury may be insensitive to the needs of his partner—which can result in a loss of intimacy.
- Because of the lack of inhibiting restraints, people with TBI must be retrained in appropriate sexual behavior. As an example, it is not unusual for a severely injured patient to masturbate in public.

---

sexual restraint (adding to the forms of inappropriate behaviors that a TBI patient may be prone to engaging in). In addition, the "ardor fodder" is mainly in the hypothalamus, that small pea-sized part of the brain that regulates temperature, metabolism, and sex drive. When the hypothalamus is damaged, it can contribute to either an abnormally high sexual drive or an extremely low one.

In some people, damage to the hypothalamus (or its partner, the pituitary gland) results in a drop in the production of the sex hormones. In others, the damaged screening mechanisms of the frontal lobes contribute to the problem by compromising the patient's judgment about sexual matters, including what, where, and, of course, when, in addition to when enough is enough. Secondary symptoms of TBI, such as depression or mania, anxiety, or increased stress, can also cause sexual dysfunction.

Some of the ways sexual dysfunction appears in TBI are:

- *Increased libido.* About 50 percent of people who have TBI have increased interest in sex and are easily sexually aroused, regardless of the circumstances surrounding that arousal.

- *Reduced libido.* About 25 percent report less sexual drive than before. (And about 25 percent report no change.)
- *Erectile dysfunction or impotence.* Approximately 40 to 60 percent of men who have TBI will experience erectile dysfunction, at least temporarily, and because it is often caused by structural damage to the brain, the medications that those of us who watch television commercials are so familiar with may be of no benefit to them.
- *Inability to reach orgasm.* Approximately 40 percent of both men and women with TBI have difficulties with sexual satisfaction.
- *Reduced frequency.* In addition to the biological damage in the brain, depression, and lack of confidence, a physical disability can make the act itself just physically uncomfortable, or a medicine can contribute to "I have a headache" tonight.
- *Role confusion.* The rhythms of the past sexual life are gone—both for the TBI victim and his or her partner. Often, following serious brain injury, the spouse needs to assume a new role of authority in the home. These new roles and rules can create anger, frustration, and alienation in both partners.

KEEPING SCORE

The effect of TBI on William T. was a heightened sex drive coupled with short-term memory loss. Several months after he'd been discharged from post-acute rehabilitation, he and his wife came to my office. She was in tears. Her husband wanted sex all the time, but just minutes after they would have sex, he would forget that they had! Consequently, he was insatiable and kept after her all the time.

I suggested they keep a chalkboard in the bedroom. Whenever they had sex, they were to tally it, and he'd have to initial it. This way, his wife could point to the board and tell her husband, "Look, we just had sex an hour ago!" so he'd leave her alone. At first, he would give in only reluctantly, but with acceptance of the finality of the decision. Once he learned that "no" meant "no," this behavioral strategy helped William regulate his impulses. The couple's sex life improved, at least from her perspective, within a few weeks.

Sexual dysfunction is not just a problem in the bedroom. It can hinder a brain-injured person's reentry into the community. When a single man with TBI, for example, acts sexually aggressive in a bar, he'll hear, "Get lost!" A brain-injured woman, on the other hand, may become easy prey because of her poor impulse-control, impaired judgment, and low self-esteem. Being an aggressor or a victim brings rejection and pain to the person with TBI—leading to even lower self-esteem.

Then there's the problem of perception found in many people with TBI. They don't think there's anything off-putting about them—even though they haven't showered in days, combed their hair, or put on clean clothes. They can't understand why they can't connect.

"THE DOWNWARD SPIRAL": DEPRESSION

People with TBI are far more likely than members of the general population to develop clinically significant depression. Several studies show that over 50 percent suffer from depression in the first year following their brain injuries. The highest rate of depression is found among those who have mild brain injuries, nearly 75 percent of whom report experiencing depression during the first year of disability. (According to the World Health Organization, among the general population only 5.8 percent of men and 9.5 percent of women will experience a depressive episode in any given year.)

These are sobering statistics, but they make sense from both a physical and psychological perspective. The denial, injury to specific parts of the brain (particularly the very front of the left frontal lobe), the pain, the disorientation, the frustration about one's limitations, the enormous changes in every aspect of one's life—it's no wonder so many TBI patients get depressed! The good news is that depression is usually temporary and can often be treated successfully.

Because depression occurs in response to chronic stress, even in those without ABI or TBI, it makes sense that those who are vulnerable to this condition will be at greater risk following such an injury. Given the despair and frustration of trying to reintegrate into normal life, it is understandable that depression would be so prevalent among the members of this group. As one of my patients said, "It's not fair. I didn't ask to be brain-injured!"

Furthermore, it has been shown that when the anterior areas particularly of the left frontal lobe are damaged by injury or stroke, a cascade of neurochemical dysfunction can take place that leads to depression in many patients, even those without a genetic predisposition to depression.

Depression may be fueled further by the rejection that occurs because the person with TBI is "different." His friends and acquaintances will likely recite a litany of complaints: "He stares at me blankly." "He's, well, dirty." "I wish he'd wash his hair." "He comes out with this outrageous stuff in the middle of class." "He's not the Johnny I knew." Not everyone can handle the changes; it's not a failing on anyone's part, it's just the reality.

Friends can lose their patience as things never seem to return to normal. Family members, unable to hide their own unhappiness and impatience, stop coming by to visit. Classmates look the other way. Jobs are lost—or never found. And spouses, ill-prepared for the life changes that TBI has brought into their routines, file for divorce. Studies show that 50 percent of marriages or partnerships fail in the first two years after the traumatic brain injury, and the statistics are even higher for those very recently married before the accident.

Many patients with TBI become so despondent and frustrated that they turn to alcohol, drugs, or inappropriate attention-seeking behavior— wearing sexually provocative clothes to work, crying on the job, or shouting out curses in class.

The solution? Therapy and the appropriate use of medications, which should start as soon as the first symptoms appear. A safe, supportive, and consistent environment will do wonders for a TBI patient's self-esteem and confidence. At our clinic, psychosocial therapy is part of every aspect of rehabilitation, as well as a separate element in a treatment plan. (We will look at different types of psychosocial therapies in Chapter 13.)

There is one more factor in TBI that must still be mentioned. It is the culmination of all these physical, cognitive, and psychosocial deficits. It is the whole that is greater than its parts, the changed personality, the alien self— the most elusive and the most critical factor of all—and it is discussed in the next chapter.

chapter 8

How TBI Can Affect Personality: The Alien Self

My today's self perpetually slips out of any hold of it that I may try to take.
—Gilbert Ryle

"Where's my family?"

"I'm still me. I think."

"No one knows me anymore."

"I feel fine, what's wrong with you?"

"Who am I?"

"What's wrong with me?"

"I feel different."

I've heard these statements and questions over and over again. From family members of people with brain injuries. From their friends and lovers. From brain-injured patients themselves. And even now, after twenty-five years as a neuropsychiatrist, they still get to me. These expressions of the loss of an individual's sense of self and irretrievable hopes for the future are still the hardest to hear.

Scientists hold various theories and assumptions about what gives us our "humanness." Never mind the research, the countless studies, the carefully tabulated statistics—all of us intuitively know that an electro-chemical reaction or a genetic predisposition falls short of defining the self; there is still the missing link between stimulus and response that makes each of us uniquely human. When someone is brain injured, that personal-ity, that essence, along with other brain functions, is disrupted.

If an adult becomes blind, it is indeed a tragedy. But after a period of ad-justment, therapy, and rehabilitation, she will learn to cope with her dis-ability. As with nearly all disabilities or illnesses, the individual's mind creates a coping strategy that she will execute over time to compensate for lost physical or sensory abilities and gradually become herself again. This is also true for many brain-injury survivors: New learning and compensatory strategies evolve as their brains go through the various stages of recovery and as new neuronal connections develop. As these adaptations consoli-date, tasks that required relearning return to being habits that no longer require so much mental or physical energy.

Sadly, for those with the severest of brain injuries, there may not be the residual brain capacity for such an outcome to be biologically possible. Al-though the blind adult can no longer see, her noninjured brain permits her to still be herself; she will still have the same tastes, the same dreams, the same beliefs. Her essence, the whole that is greater than the sum of its biological parts, or, as the poets say, her soul, will still be intact. However, for a person with a severe traumatic brain injury, that essence often seems to be gone. The brain, the organ of the mind, has been hurt, and that translates into changes in the self—in behavior, perception, thinking, memory, and personality. It is that dreaded loss of self so frequently seen in literature and seen in movies that has always been portrayed as a supreme, personal violation.

Many brain-injured people, especially following severe acceleration-deceleration injuries or large strokes, lose the ability to be self-reflective, to have insight into their problems, and, most frustrating of all for those who love them, to be aware of how they've changed. On one level, this can be a blessing, because an individual who lacks self-awareness—that is, suffers from *anosognosia*—is spared the realization that his life will never be same. For the rehabilitation team and especially the survivor's family, however, facing this situation is a tremendous challenge, for such an individual is biologically unable to recognize his need for help and therefore may resist all attempts at change.

Nevertheless, progress is certainly possible, and many brain-injured people have gone on to live useful, happy lives even after losing their cognitive skills and living with physical disabilities. Their adaptations to their new lives are usually hard won, often occurring after experiencing the natural consequences that the real world doles out to each of us, regardless of disability or social status, when unexpected difficulties prevent us from normal functioning. Expectations of real reintegration back into one's community are often frustrated by the remaining reality that communities integrate those whom they choose to, despite legislative mandates that attempt to correct for some of the shortcomings in society's treatment of the disabled. Behavioral problems occurring in a community shopping mall or local restaurant are met with security or police intervention, not the empathic understanding of families or rehab teams. Friends drift away as they realize they have lost an old friend to the impact of brain injury on memory and the friend's ability to provide the reciprocity expected in true friendship.

Yet, for those survivors who persist in using the strategies they have learned in rehabilitation, new friends emerge. The brain-injured person bonds with others through new social activities. Although the type of work the TBI patient performed before the injury may no longer be possible, new jobs are often available that can accommodate his needs. Earning a paycheck enhances one's feelings of dignity, self-worth, and pride, as does performing a job successfully. These experiences are their own reward and serve to prevent the isolation that invariably comes from unemployment and the sense of failure that accompanies the inability to "pay one's own way."

THE NEW JOHN

A new self for John Stambino, a thirty-one-year-old musician, was born in an act of senseless violence in 2000, when he and his band buddies went to a convenience store to get some snacks before they went to play at a club. They were in the store when a gunman wearing a ski mask came in with a loaded .38 semiautomatic. When the clerk did not respond fast enough to demands for cash, the gunman started shooting; he killed five people and injured several more before killing himself. One of John's band members was killed and John was severely injured when he was shot in the head. He survived his injury and was taken to a nearby trauma center for treatment.

John lay in a coma for six days. His new life began with a series of operations that led to the loss of three-quarters of his right frontal lobe. Then came the residual symptoms of his gunshot wound: the inability to walk, the crying that wouldn't stop, the loss of memory. Widespread damage to the right side of his brain where the bullet exited his skull left him incapable of sensing the left side of his body. When he later learned how to shave again, he would shave only half his face; he didn't recognize the other half as being his face.

As his strength returned, John became obsessive-compulsive. He continually felt compelled to wash his hands, and he had to have everything ordered in a certain way. For example, he insisted on keeping nine of every item that he used in his daily activities, believing that if his world was held together by his lucky number his anxiety would decrease. When he could walk again, he had to go up and down the stairs literally nine times before he felt comfortable leaving the house; he had to count to nine before taking a bite of food, and he had to brush each region of his teeth nine times before going to bed. If he didn't, his anxiety escalated to the point where he couldn't contain it; the obsessive-compulsive disorder (OCD) led him to believe that something horrible would happen to his parents or to him if these rules were not followed.

"I know I'm different," he said. "But who cares? I can still get the job done." Unfortunately, he had many different jobs after leaving acute rehab: He could get jobs, but keeping them was an entirely different matter. John could follow workplace rules, but he could not always correctly understand them or manage to generalize a specific situation to more general patterns of behavior. And, of course, his stacked rows could only contain nine items in any one stack.

Besides the OCD, John had continual difficulties with impulse control. When his mother explained to him why he couldn't do or say certain things—why he couldn't scream at people, for example—John felt bad, often saying over and over again that he really didn't mean to do it. But he missed the connection between action and its regulation by thought, instead responding with his first impulses. He often had to be bluntly told that he was acting inappropriately, as he just couldn't objectively realize that his actions were disruptive to others. Of course, he was remorseful, but he truly did not realize the impact of his behavior on others. He never planned to be disruptive; it was just what happened when he felt an emotional impulse and expressed it without conscious thought as to its consequences.

After coming to terms with his repeated failures, John was determined to get better and, for a brief, shining moment in time, it looked like he would. A year after leaving his first rehabilitation facility, John reunited with his uninjured band members and two new players to perform at a well-known rock club in New York City, where they put on a benefit concert to help raise money for John's rehabilitation. He played his guitar, a skill that he had retained despite his other deficits, as his prior motor memory in this area was unaffected. Once he got into the groove and no longer had to think about what he was doing, he really began to rock, and the crowd went wild. As the band concluded its performance by playing "We Are the Champions," people began dancing in the aisles, singing along, feeling the miracle of the John they used to know seemingly restored.

But the dream was shattered only two weeks later. During a band rehearsal, John had a severe seizure associated with flashing lights and fell from the stage, striking his head, and had to be rushed to the ER. His hopes of returning to his old life were crushed that day as the second brain injury only compounded the effects of the gunshot wound. His once intermittent seizure disorder became extremely unstable, risking his safety. Furthermore, it had become apparent that John was incapable of performing the executive functions involved in leading a band, such as making performance dates, organizing shows, and more, and he irrationally lashed out at others when they disagreed with him. This wasn't the John his friends and family had known. There was no going back. The band dissolved.

You can still feel the sensitivity of an artist in John despite his cognitive and behavioral disabilities. He doesn't retain the memories of the person he was prior to his injuries, but a part of him will always dream of that boy who, he has been told, was the student-body president of his high school, sang in a rock band, and had such a bright future ahead of him brimming with the hope of youthful exuberance and invincibility.

Like other traumatically brain-injured people whose executive functions are impaired, John's symptoms demonstrated his inability to reflect on his own behavior and learn from the feedback given to him by others. Other symptoms associated with his dysfunctional obsessiveness, impulsiveness, and lack of empathy would have escalated if his family had not obtained guardianship of his affairs to protect him from his poor judgment and, specifically, from being exploited by others because of it. After assuming guardianship, his family exercised their court-appointed rights to readmit him to a well-established post-acute residential brain-injury center, despite his initial objections that he was "just fine and didn't need any help."

Without a return to a therapeutic environment, in all likelihood his deficits would have continued to worsen, risking his safety or the safety of others; he may have even ended up in jail during one of his out-of-control public displays. Without treatment, the confusion of his thought processes and his inability to concentrate, focus, or plan could have continued to worsen. As it was, his anger had reached the point where he would explode with little or no provocation. His lack of control would intensify before eventually burning itself out as he became more and more fatigued. Unfortunately, these handicaps are quite common following severe brain injuries and tend to worsen with time. Holding the line with a thirty-something-year-old man can be very difficult when his behavioral deregulation becomes increasingly fixed as a part of his handicap. Parents, partners, friends—and even the family doctor—usually have little experience with this level of dyscontrol and unwittingly come to accept it as just a part of their new lives.

It's often hard for people to accept that injuries to the brain can have such catastrophic effects on a person's personality and mind; friends and even family members of a brain-injured person often believe that the troublesome behavior of their loved one is all just a reaction to his changed circumstances and that he will get back to normal as he "grows out of it." This is wishful thinking. At some point, the last straw will break the back of a family system, forcing all concerned to recognize that despite the time elapsed since the original injuries, treatment is necessary to help reestablish some normalcy. Returning to treatment may be taken as a personal failure by the family, yet it is the only reasonable option when life has become an unrelenting series of crises.

Of course, electing to intervene is no easy task; often families experience guilt born of the sense of failure and despair that accompanies a problem that just can't be cured. John remained in his new treatment program for over a year, and during that time, with all the resources of a secure environment and an experienced interdisciplinary rehabilitation team working in his favor, his behavioral control improved. His OCD and depression responded to appropriate medications, and he became engaged in activities that provided him with a series of small successes that helped to rebuild his self-esteem and instill in him a desire to change, despite his difficulties in recognizing what actually had to change within himself. He gradually had therapeutic assignments with his family, at first in the neighboring community and then back at home, where he practiced behavioral strategies designed to help him psychically recognize when his anxiety or irritability began to escalate—before it got out of control.

THE NEW EMILY

For my patient Emily Carter, who had dreamed of a career in broadcasting but suffered a severe head injury in a car accident at the age of eighteen, the difficulties were different from those experienced by John Stambino. The members of the treatment team have come to know her and her family very well, as she recently entered her sixteenth year under my care as her attending physician. Emily experienced a number of troubling symptoms in the early phases of her recovery, including a prolonged mutism—she struggled with initiating any speech whatsoever. Fortunately, she responded to treatment when the medication bromocriptine (Parlodel) was given to her.

Now, she just can't seem to stop talking, and although the frequency of our visits has varied over the years, depending on her needs, we have dealt with many of the life issues that any young woman in her situation would face as she matured.

Emily's personality changes were never as apparent as those exhibited by John. However, as the reality of losing all of her high school friends set in—as they moved on in their lives and graduated from college—she began to gain weight. It didn't help that she remained out of shape and lacked the motivation to sustain an exercise program and prescribed diet for weight control. Her diminished self-awareness prevented her from describing her feelings as those of depression, and she reported that her mood was "just fine." But she showed all the classic symptoms of depression: loss of enjoyment of previously enjoyable experiences, sleeping ten hours a day, and a weight increase of twenty pounds over three months. Plus, she showed evidence of irritability each morning. Luckily, she responded extremely well to cognitive behavioral therapy (CBT) and the antidepressant medication paroxetine. These treatments led to a complete resolution of her symptoms within two months.

However, as she began to feel and look better, her risk-taking behavior increased, and she began "clubbing" every weekend. Given her intolerance of alcohol, she was an easy target for predatory young men. This led to her getting pregnant and having to make an agonizing decision about whether she could manage caring for a baby when so much of her day was spent taking care of her own needs.

Ultimately, she decided to have her child, despite the fact that the father had vanished—she never saw him again. Her executive dysfunction made it difficult for her to care for her child. Tragically, she also has trouble expressing empathy, as this emotion is the product of an intact prefrontal cortex, and this deficit made it difficult for her and the child to closely bond. She is more like a friend to her daughter than a mother. In these circumstances, she is fortunate that her own mother has been a constant source of support. In fact, she bought Emily a home next door to her own so as to have a regular presence in her daughter's and granddaughter's lives.

As time progressed, Emily continued to undergo treatment for her depression and took parenting classes that taught her skills to compensate for those deficits that made parenting difficult for her. As of this writing, Emily still lives next door to her mother and works part-time as a courier for her mother's day-care centers. She is even able to drive a car safely. She has learned to be a good mother and is delighted that she made the decision to keep her daughter. Her job gives her time to be by herself and meet her own needs while earning some money for the extra things she wants for her daughter.

Is she the Emily who wanted to go into broadcasting? No. Is she the Emily who dreamed of adventure under the big lights? No. But she *is* Emily Carter, a mother and woman who is enthusiastic, happy, and proud of what she has accomplished, despite leading a very different kind of life than the one she had planned when she was in high school.

This is it. The damage has been done and discussed. It's time now to talk about returning, of rehabilitation that works, of a world after TBI.

Life is waiting.

PART 3

TREATING TBI:
FROM ER THROUGH REHAB

chapter 9

EMERGENCY AND
ACUTE CARE

> *To enhance public awareness of the benefits to*
> *be derived from brain research, the Congress, by*
> *House Joint Resolution 174, has designated the*
> *decade beginning January 1, 1990, as the*
> *"Decade of the Brain" and has authorized and*
> *requested the President to issue a proclamation*
> *in observance of this occasion. . . . As a first*
> *priority we must ensure access to specialized*
> *neurotrauma centers, which have proven to*
> *save lives.*
> —Office of the Federal Register,
> July 18, 1990

In an ideal world, the ambulance would come racing to the scene, or the medevac chopper would appear overhead at the location of an accident, within minutes after it occurred. The head-injury victim would be rushed to a neurotrauma center where initial evaluation and treatment would immediately begin.

Before the victim was even moved from the scene of the accident, the emergency medical technicians (EMTs) would triage the situation, perform CPR, and intubate his trachea with a breathing tube to ensure that oxygen could get to the lungs. They would stabilize his neck in case there was also an injury to his spinal cord, to prevent permanent compression, and apply tourniquets to any hemorrhaging limbs. Next, the patient would be placed on a backboard and put into the ambulance. Here, intravenous fluids (IVs) would be started, the patient's heart would be monitored with an EKG, and the hospital would be alerted about his current status, including his initial Glasgow Coma Scale score, and emergency medications would be started upon the recommendation of a physician.

Upon arrival at the hospital or Level I Trauma Center, more in-depth testing would begin to clarify the initial severity of the patient's condition and look for evolving life-threatening complications. Blood would be drawn and tested to see if it was being adequately oxygenated. A screening neurological examination would be done to look for signs suggestive of increased intracranial pressure or cranial nerve entrapment. The rest of his body would be examined for other injuries that may also be life-threatening, especially internal bleeding. If needed, brain and abdominal CT scans would be performed to look for bleeding or the suggestion of increased intracranial pressure or brain displacement. If any significant abnormalities were seen, neurosurgeons and general surgeons would be consulted. Together, the physicians would evaluate the need for surgical intervention, whether to remove an epidural hematoma or repair a lacerated liver.

THE ROLE OF SURGERY

When a loved one has a traumatic brain injury, family members and friends see a gurney rushed to a trauma unit, the doors quickly closing behind the crew of EMTs, and physicians and nurses going into action. They hope that somehow the doctors will work miracles behind those closed doors—that somehow the surgeons will put their loved one back together so that he will be as good as new. But when the types of brain injury that are the focus of this book occur, they happen very rapidly, leaving damaged tissue where moments earlier there was healthy tissue.

Neurosurgery is almost always performed within the first hours or days after a TBI. However, because TBI has no exact pattern, there is no set rule. Basically, surgery for TBI has three main goals:

1. To save a life
2. To prevent initial damage from getting worse
3. To prevent foreseeable complications from becoming life-threatening

There are four common reasons for surgery after TBI. They are:
1. To remove blood clots (hematomas)
2. To ease pressure on the brain from swelling
3. To stop bleeding
4. To repair skull fractures

Let's look at each of the four situations more closely.

Removing Blood Clots, or Hematomas

The most immediately life-threatening type of traumatic brain injury occurs when the skull is fractured and a major artery, the *middle meningeal artery,* is ruptured by the shards of the collapsed bone.

When this occurs, the artery continues to pump blood into the space between the skull and the dural covering of the brain. As this clot, or hematoma, expands, it forces the brain to displace the structures located beneath it into other brain compartments that force the brain downward toward the cerebellum and foramen magnum.

The life-sustaining parts of the brain stem and cerebellum are then forced (*herniated*) into the spinal canal, where they are compressed. Within minutes, as blood supply is also blocked by compression, a brain injury victim can die. This type of hematoma requires immediate neurosurgical intervention to save the patient's life. The surgery involves opening the scalp and removing the bones surrounding the fracture in order to expose the clot. The clot is then taken out, and the middle meningeal artery is tied off at each broken end in order to stop further bleeding.

The other common type of hematoma is a *subdural hematoma,* which occurs when the supporting blood vessels between the dura and arachnoid are torn, often as a result of the rapid deceleration of the skull. These vessels are veins, which bleed more slowly than arteries, making this situation more insidious than the arterial rupture described above.

When any body structure or part of an organ is abnormally forced into a part of the body where it does not belong, this movement is termed a herniation. A "hernia," for example, occurs when part of the small intestine is forced through a ring in the groin and moves into the testicles. Similarly, when the brain is forced into foreign compartments, there are several resulting herniation syndromes that may develop. Neurosurgical removal is often required to prevent herniation; however, if the subdural hematoma is small and does not appear to be expanding, a "watch and wait" path may be chosen to prevent the risks associated with surgically opening the skull and removing the dura to evacuate the clot.

Acceleration and then deceleration of the head (such as typically occurs in a car accident) may also produce hematomas that need surgical intervention. In this case the force of impact creates a situation in which the skull is fractured while the brain continues to move within it. This can occur in a coup-contrecoup injury.

If the bruising, or *contusion*, of the brain is particularly severe, surgery will usually be performed to remove the blood and parts of the brain that are irrevocably damaged and that if left in the brain will swell to the point of producing life-threatening herniation syndromes.

When the blood clot that develops within the structure of the brain is caused by the rupture of an internal blood vessel, however, the call for surgery is much more complicated.

As you can imagine, surgical removal of a clot in a functional part of the brain, termed an *intracerebral hematoma*, may add insult to injury. There is just no way to avoid destroying living brain tissue, as removing the clot involves also removing some viable brain tissue surrounding it. Once again, the risks are always weighed against the larger danger that an expanding clot may cause death.

Easing Pressure on the Brain

When you bruise your knee or your ankle, the tissue underneath the skin can swell. Similarly, a TBI can make the bruised brain swell (causing *edema*). But, just as in the case of a hematoma, the brain has nowhere to go; it can only swell so much before it reaches the limited capacity of the skull to permit this type of expansion. The swelling then exerts pressure on the brain, squeezing it to the point where cells die and parts of the brain are displaced into areas where there is no room to accommodate them. This *intracranial pressure (ICP)*, by compressing both arteries and veins, can prevent blood from properly circulating in the brain, resulting in even more brain-cell damage.

Increased ICP is considered among the most dangerous results of a TBI. Studies show that the buildup of pressure from an injury can cause more secondary damage than a hematoma. The good news is that often the pressure does not reach life-threatening levels and, with time, generally subsides to normal, preinjury levels. The bad news? A few hours of excess pressure can cause irreparable damage, in part because it compromises total brain blood flow. Increased ICP must be closely monitored.

In non-life-threatening cases, that monitoring is best done by inserting an ICP monitor through the skull to rest on the brain so that physicians can have a continuous reading of the intracranial pressure. If the monitor shows increased pressure, they can immediately administer medications to help lower it. If severe, sustained increases do not respond to medications, neurosurgery is often done in which the surgeon removes the entire skullcap to provide room for the brain to expand without compromising its viability. Once the pressure subsides, the skull (*calvaria*) is replaced and the scalp is stitched back together, preventing permanent disfigurement.

Sometimes there is a buildup of cerebrospinal fluid, the fluid that surrounds the brain; as it circulates, it may fill up the spaces, or ventricles, between certain brain structures. This condition is called *hydrocephalus*, and it, too, can create dangerous pressure on the brain. If this buildup of fluid is caused by a blockage of its outflow to the spinal column, usually as the result of bleeding (*intraventricular hemorrhage*), surgery must be performed to insert a shunt (or tube) into the brain to drain the fluid into the abdomen. This procedure is called placement of an *intraventricular shunt*.

Stopping Internal Bleeding, or Hemorrhaging

Another cause of an immediate brain injury is a ruptured *aneurysm*. Surgery is often indicated in these cases as well. Although not always a result

Brain surgery is the oldest type of medical procedure. Archaeological evidence shows that it was performed even during prehistoric times. Although scientists can only speculate about why such procedures were performed, there is radiographic evidence within the patterns of the skulls discovered by archaeologists to suggest that they were performed to release pressure on the brain. Where no such residual imaging evidence is found, it is presumed that surgery was performed to "release evil humors," either to help people with presumed neuropsychiatric conditions or as part of sacrificial rites.

of trauma to the brain, an aneurysm, like a stroke, can occur because of a weakness in one of the arterial blood vessels. This weakness eventually forces a vulnerable area of the blood vessel, usually at the junction where two vessels come together, to balloon out. Eventually, the weakened wall of the ballooned area can no longer take the constant pumping pressure produced by the healthy arteries, and it breaks, or ruptures. In this situation, a neurosurgeon may need to go into the brain, find the ballooned area of the damaged blood vessel, and "clip" it to stop the bleeding. This is a high-risk procedure, but it may be necessary if the doctor determines that the patient may not survive without it. In these circumstances, one must choose the lesser of two evils. By choosing surgery, the doctor prevents certain death.

Repairing Skull Fractures

Just like the bones of the arms, legs, and hips, the skull can break, or fracture, in an accident. Unfortunately, a skull fracture, especially one that gets depressed inward as the result of an external force, can leave bits of bone embedded in the brain tissue. These fragments must be removed and the skull repaired to prevent further brain damage. Surgical intervention may also be needed to prevent further pressure from developing in the brain tissue beneath the fracture. Finally, fractures can also cause an arterial rupture like that seen with an epidural hematoma.

IT *Is* BRAIN SURGERY

In order to repair the brain, a neurosurgeon must be able to get to it. Sounds simple, right? In reality, several very complex procedures are involved.

1. The head is shaved and a scalp incision is made in the area where the damage is most extensive. The scalp is retracted from the bone of the skull.

2. A craniotomy is performed next as a piece of skull is cut off and put aside. It will usually be replaced after the brain surgery has been completed. If there is extensive skull damage, such as shattered fragments or multiple fractures, the flap will not be replaced. In this situation, titanium or hardened plastic plates will be placed over the brain to protect it from further injury.

3. The exposed dural membrane is also carefully cut.

4. Now the brain surgery can be performed. Any hematomas are removed. Bits of bone are taken out. Hemorrhaging is stopped. A bleeding aneurysm (in the case of a stroke) is repaired (clipped). An ICP monitor is inserted, if necessary.

5. When possible, the dura is carefully sutured back over the brain.

6. The skull flap is replaced. If there is severe swelling, a surgeon may wait a few weeks before replacing it, until the swelling (edema) has gone down.

WATCHING AND WAITING AS THE BRAIN HEALS

Once the brain has been severely damaged, it continues to suffer the consequences of an avalanche of physical and chemical events for hours to days following the initial trauma. At present there is little that medicine can do to prevent the consequences of the evolving biochemical difficulties, but since the advent of neurotrauma centers, rapid neurosurgical intervention has saved tens of thousands of lives that would have been lost just two decades ago. Following the surgical interventions described above, appropriate medical treatments are started to support life until the brain begins to heal. The patient's next treatment landmark is placement in an intensive care unit, where the focus shifts from immediate intervention to watching and waiting.

This is a difficult phase for both families and treatment teams because it's too early to be certain that a severely injured individual will survive, though the immediate fear of death is over. Always wanting to have a family prepared for the worst, neurosurgeons are, usually for good reasons, pessimistic when discussing prognosis with the family whose loved one is in the early phases of ICU care. If the person dies, at least everyone was prepared; if he doesn't, there are no complaints. The watching and waiting are necessary steps of the recovery process because there is very little that medical science can do to speed it along at this stage. Efforts are directed at preventing secondary complications from developing that may further endanger the patient's survival. Things like rising intracranial pressure, the development of pneumonia, and erratic autonomic responses all have the potential to disrupt recovery. Vigilant care providers begin treatment at the earliest signs of a complication to lessen its impact on recovery and prevent it from becoming life-threatening.

With the passage of time, the body as well as the mind begins to stabilize and the patient can be weaned from the ventilator. The scans can be done less frequently, and the various monitoring devices—such as those initially needed for constant evaluation of ICP; oxygen saturation of the blood; telemetric measurements based on EKGs of the heart, including blood pressure and heart rate; and ventilator settings—are gradually reduced in number. At this stage, a patient is transferred from the intensive care setting to a step-down unit where monitoring still regularly occurs, but with less intensity.

If all goes well, the patient may soon be able to respond to the environment and be ready for the physical challenges of therapy. When her level of arousal increases and she is able to benefit from rehabilitative services, she will be transferred to an acute rehabilitation hospital.

The period of time that it takes to reach this stage varies widely depending on the severity of the injury. In a mild injury, the period of unconsciousness is so brief that the person usually arrives at the hospital in a somewhat responsive state. Posttraumatic amnesia lasts only minutes to an hour, and retrograde amnesia is generally so fleeting as to be unnoticeable. Confusion and agitation are mild, and there are no deficits in the person's ability to perform her usual ADLs and function within the confines of a quiet environment. If the injury is very mild and surgery was not necessary, inpatient rehabilitation may not be necessary; instead, recovery can take place in outpatient settings. If the injury is more severe, the transition to acute rehab may not occur for days, weeks, or months. Often acute care hospitals will transfer the patient to a specialty medical hospital with an established neurorehabilitative team before the patient is ready for acute rehab. Such transfers free up needed beds at the acute care hospital and permit the next level of care to occur in an environment that is less stressful for the patient and family. The specialty medical hospital is an intermediate stage between the acute care hospital and the more intensive rehabilitation services that can be provided in an acute rehab hospital.

THE SPECIALTY MEDICAL HOSPITAL

For slow-to-recover patients, admission to a specialty medical hospital (SMH) permits a more prolonged period of recovery to occur. Patients in this category may have remained in a coma for some time. They may not have opened their eyes or experienced the return of a normalized sleep-wake cycle for a month, and then may have remained in a vegetative or minimally responsive state for an additional period of time. During this stage, the patient's eyes open spontaneously and periods of sleep alternating with episodes of apparent wakefulness return, signaling that a relatively normal sleep-wake cycle has been restored. Technically, when these two neurologic abilities return, a person is no longer considered in "true coma." However, these individuals cannot yet participate in the programs and therapies offered in acute rehab hospitals. The central nervous system has yet to come online to make new learning possible.

For these patients, the neurospecialty team of the SMH picks up where the intensive care or step-down units of the acute care hospital leave off. In some cases, when patients have been on ventilators for breathing support, they must be weaned off of them very gradually as the brain begins to heal naturally. It is rarely possible to just abruptly stop ventilator support; instead, patients are given progressively longer times off of it, without the removal of the tracheotomy, or the tube initially placed into the trachea (or windpipe), until the treatment team is confident that the patient can breathe on his own. Furthermore, a patient must be turned every two hours by trained staff members to prevent skin breakdown caused by the patient's inability to move. Turning the patient relieves pressure on the skin, especially on the buttocks.

In this setting, the focus on preventing secondary complications intensifies as the brain slowly continues to recover. Progress seems subtle, and time frames elongated. As an example, once a patient opens her eyes, the first sign of progress is usually that she begins tracking the movement of people in her environment with her eyes; however, she will remain mute. Physical therapy is initiated, but it is more passive than active. The therapist will work on providing stretching exercises designed to prevent the development of *contractures*, that is, the tightening of muscles, tendons, ligaments, or skin that restricts normal movement of a limb or the neck. In severely brain-injured patients, contractures develop in response to prolonged posturing that occurs as a result of specific lesions (abnormalities) in parts of the brain controlling muscle movement. (See Chapter 5 for more information about abnormal posturing.)

In cases of severe posturing, where the risk of developing permanent contractures is greatest, the therapist will fit the patient for special splints designed to counteract the abnormal tone. The medical team decides if a trial of an intrathecal baclofen pump is warranted to help reduce the posturing even further, permitting increased comfort for the patient and greater ease in repositioning him to prevent skin breakdown.

Since the patient cannot swallow, feeding occurs following a percutaneous endoscopic gastrostomy (PEG), a procedure that involves inserting a tube directly into the stomach so that needed fluid, calories, and nutrients may be administered to the patient via a pump. This tube is also used for the administration of most medications. It often surprises people to realize how many calories a person actually needs even when he looks as though he is in a state of suspended animation.

With appropriate care, very gradually many patients start to respond to the environment around them, become capable of following simple commands, and eventually begin to speak. As these changes occur, the neurospecialty team increases the amount of therapy done with the patient each day. Rather than having this therapy occur over an entire hour, it is usually broken up into multiple segments of fifteen minutes each. This helps a person with a short attention span, who becomes easily fatigued, receive the maximum benefit from her therapy time rather than wasting three-fourths of it.

At this juncture, some patients are ready to begin acute rehabilitation. Depending on the availability of local resources and the experience of the individuals who make up the rehab team, this transition may occur at the SMH; in other situations, the patient is transferred to a separate acute rehabilitation hospital or a specialized residential brain-injury program.

chapter 10

REHABILITATION 101

Time is brain.
—Anonymous

The road is deserted. I turn on my stereo and start singing along to my favorite CD. I open the window on the driver's side to let in the fresh, cool air. I'm coasting. I feel magically transported back to my teenage years, driving my hot wheels, not a care in the world. It feels good. I go a little faster. Why not? No one's around. The light changes to green ahead of me. I don't want to have to wait for it to turn red again. I pull a little faster into the intersection, still singing, still smiling, as a truck enters from the right. I see it out of the corner of my eye. I honk the horn. He has a red light. What is he doing? It's too late. "Stop!" I scream as the truck crashes into the passenger side of my car. Suddenly, I'm spinning, around and around, and then . . .

I wake up on a table, a light glaring over me. There are people all around, wearing masks and aprons. My eyes hurt. They are pushing and prodding me. Where am I? What's going on? I try to turn, but I can't. My head's in some kind of vise. I try to kick the strangers away, but then they're all on top of me and I can't move again. I'm about to lose my mind—can't seem to get a grip. Something comes out of my mouth, but who knows what it means. All I can feel is pain.

I can't remember much of anything except the glare of the light that hurt my eyes. They tell me I'm in a trauma center. That I had an accident. I don't know

what a trauma center is. I don't know what's going on. I'm in pain and I'm ex-
hausted. Things go black again . . .

Weeks later, I know that I was in a wreck and that I'm in a hospital, but it still
doesn't make much sense. They say I hurt my head and broke some bones, so
what does that mean? They tell me I have to be patient, that I need time to heal,
that I'll need some kind of rehab. My family's here, my wife looks worried, she
holds my hand a lot. Somehow, the rest of the family has shown up, even my kid
brother. They visit a lot, but what is there to say? I just want to go home, but they
say I have to stay, maybe even go to another hospital. All I really need is to get
back to work. They say, "Don't worry about money," that they'll take care of that.
What a line! They never had a nickel to their names. They must be nuts.

Well, no matter what I say, I'm not going home; they're sending me to another
money-grubbing hospital. Some doctor who doesn't look old enough to shave is
acting like he's in charge. What a joke! I still can't remember what happened to
me, but who cares; I've done my time, I'm ready to go home. Now, I've got a new
cast of characters bugging me. For god's sake, why can't they just leave me alone?
One of them says she's a physical therapist, but I'll tell you what she is, she's a
physical terrorist. All the bending and stretching. Can't she get it through her
thick skull that it hurts?

Again, all I hear from those bright, smiling faces, fresh from their beds at
home, is to try to calm down—that I need time to heal. What can they know?
They're barely old enough to be out of high school. I've got responsibilities—a
family to take care of. They try to be my "friends." Well, I don't need any more
friends, and I wouldn't choose these characters if they were the last people on
earth. So, what am I going to do? I feel weird, like I'm not really me. But my
baby-faced doctor tells me that's not unusual. So what is usual?

At least I can get to the toilet by myself again—maybe some of this nonsense
just might help. I guess I'll give it one chance tomorrow. What else have I got to
do anyway?

The fictional narrator speaking about his experience shows the confusion
and frustration of a typical brain-injured person who is just coming to terms
with what has happened to him. You can sense his lack of understanding of

his need for help and rehabilitation, but then the beginning of the realization that maybe there is some usefulness to the exercises he is being asked to perform. Rehabilitation from brain injury is a slow and sometimes painful process.

Traumatic brain injury instantaneously changes a person's life and the lives of those he loves. Most likely there will be both physical and mental deficits. Without early and competent rehabilitation, these deficits will become more and more a part of the pattern of how a person functions, making them more difficult to overcome later on. Instead of relearning basic skills, the "I" in this story could have become a hopeless case, living a shadow life or worse. A dangerous cycle begins with that calamitous event, regardless of its cause, and it may change a person forever, especially if he is not taken under the wing of an experienced team that recognizes his limitations but insists that he can do more despite them.

REHAB FIRST STEPS

Rehabilitation is designed to help a person with TBI remediate as many of his residual strengths as possible during recovery and develop skills and compensatory strategies so she can live as independently as possible. As the patient relearns the skills of daily life, the burden of care for her family is reduced and she begins to obtain the best possible quality of life. We will look at some case studies to see how the post-acute rehabilitation process works out for some individual patients; but first, some general remarks about these settings are in order.

In an acute rehab setting, the pace of activity and the diversity of therapy both increase. At this point, the medical team and the physical therapist are joined by others: the occupational therapists, who, despite their title, generally focus on the rehabilitation of the upper extremities; speech and language pathologists, who help the patient with any speech deficits that have resulted from the injury; recreational therapists, who can help to integrate many of the therapies into enjoyable activities that can be rehearsed over and over again without seeming like therapy; and psychologists, both those specializing in counseling and those more focused on assessing and improving an individual's cognitive skills, helping the patient adapt to both her emotional experiences and her changed thought processes.

Generally, these activities occur within a very structured day that provides for specified periods of rest. Physicians still manage the overall status of the patient, while nurses form the backbone of the team with their around-the-clock expertise. Team conferences are held at which representatives from the entire team have an opportunity to discuss a patient's progress (or lack thereof) and plan for the introduction of new strategies designed to reduce residual handicaps.

As time goes on and the patient progresses, families are asked to participate more in the care of their loved one by attending team conferences. This helps the family members to better understand the ongoing game plan. Family members also begin to spend time with the therapists as they work individually with the patient. This training is vital so that the transition from hospital to home can go as smoothly as possible. Ideally, the transition can be made without interrupting ongoing therapeutic progress. Family members will also play an important role in making sure the patient takes medications. At least one family member must learn how to help administer or monitor the medications and know what the possible side effects are. This family member should also understand the reasoning behind the use of each medication so he or she will know how important it is that the patient take the medications.

Before the patient is discharged, a trained therapist will actually visit the patient's home to help the family prepare for any modifications or adaptations that may need to be done to the environment before it can successfully and safely accommodate their loved one's residual disabilities. If the patient is expected to be able to drive a car, a therapist will arrange to evaluate his level of competence to resume this activity. Finally, that magical day of discharge occurs and the survivor and his family begin the next phase of recovery outside the confines of a hospital.

Some patients' demands exceed what can reasonably be accommodated by the family without a total disruption of their lives. This is where the availability of a post-acute rehabilitation center is vital to prevent a breakdown in the family, in the breadwinner's capacity to earn a living, or in a young spouse's ability to care for children while also caring for a brain-injured part-ner. A good post-acute rehabilitation center has "prosthetic" environmental modifications and tools that function much like any other prosthesis—something designed to reduce or eliminate the impact of a disability on an individual's ability to live a normal life—whether it be an artificial limb to permit walking or a wheelchair to help accomplish grocery shopping. In the case of a prosthetic environment, this means that everything is tailor-made for a person with disabilities. From metal hand-bars in the bathroom to labels on drawers, cabinets, and clothes, the center is environmentally designed and professionally staffed to provide the necessary resources to help compensate for any deficits a TBI patient may have.

The living areas and therapeutic environments of the post-acute resi-dential rehab centers are often more home-like than the formal medical settings that the patient has encountered in the acute general, special, and rehabilitation hospitals. These post-acute centers are designed to help patients adapt to the real world when they leave. Treatment is pro-vided in a safe, supervised, and consistent environment that often in-cludes a community living or family room, a therapeutic kitchen, and a laundry room—all areas where patients can, through normalized, every-day living, relearn skills and/or develop compensatory strategies to reen-ter the community. In the therapeutic kitchen, for example, both cognitive and occupational therapy are in action as patients plan meals for the week or learn how to move their hands to sort ingredients in a recipe, using adaptive equipment.

In the living room, executive function and appropriate behavior are re-inforced. Patients decide as a group where to go when they have an off-campus trip. Many such trips are organized during a patient's stay. They are designed to be real-life therapeutic activities—residents may go to a bank, a supermarket, or a restaurant, for example—all opportunities for them to relearn and practice social skills, executive functioning, and even motor skills. In the laundry room, patients are taught the necessary skills to suc-cessfully sort, wash, dry, and fold their clothes. Depending on the severity of her deficits and on her progress (which is regularly reviewed), an indi-vidual may resume complete responsibility for doing her own laundry;

others may require step-by-step, hand-over-hand assistance from the rehab staff to relearn every step of the process.

Post-acute rehabilitation programs for brain-injured individuals also may have classrooms, computer labs, and other settings specially designed to enable the patients to practice prevocational skills. There may be a greenhouse, an auto-detail shop, or a print shop, for example. These settings provide for additional therapy and can be used to teach work skills that might even be translated into employment opportunities when an individual returns home. For those who are capable of participating in group therapeutic sessions that require a return of continuous memory and declarative learning, specialized groups are led by trained therapists who focus on a variety of issues—for example, self-image concerns, anger management, and substance-abuse counseling.

In addition to providing a comfortable, home-like environment, a good post-acute rehabilitation facility thus allows patients to work on their deficits and to learn prevocational skills that will help them return to productive activity. The setting is designed to keep stress levels low as this recovery and learning take place, as well as to provide each participant with unconditional regard, regardless of his level of handicap. This does not mean that all maladaptive behaviors are acceptable—rather, it means that they are viewed in the context of an individual's residual capacities for learning. The therapeutic interventions are adapted to the person's individual needs and strengths. Redirection is not punitive; instead, it provides an appropriate context for new learning.

The brief case studies presented next demonstrate how these concepts are put into action in a post-acute setting.

CASE STUDIES: POST-ACUTE REHABILITATION

Remember Bruce Robertson, who suffered a TBI as a result of a car accident in the Nevada desert, and who now keeps a journal to help overcome his amnesia? His story was told in Chapter 6. During his post-acute rehabilitation, Bruce enjoyed working in the auto shop in our rehab center. The auto shop is designed to help patients learn basic skills focused on automobile and small-engine repair. He especially liked polishing the cars and tinkering with the small engines to make them run like new again. Embedded in the program are activities that teach important vocational skills and group cooperation while providing appropriate redirection by a "vocational supervisor." Bruce's hobby also provided him with real-life physical therapy, because as he worked he strengthened his arm muscles and improved both his range of motion and his physical endurance. Bruce is now a manager at his apartment complex, as well as an ordained minister, as noted earlier. Even though he did not turn out to be a mechanic, the auto-shop experience taught him valuable skills and lessons.

Then there is Emily Carter, who overcame depression following her accident only to become pregnant as the result of a one-night stand (described in Chapter 8). Earlier in her recovery process, she, too, was at our post-acute rehab center. In the center's print shop, after lots of practice she finally got the hang of carefully maintaining the correct amount of pressure on the silk-screening machine to print a four-color drawing on a T-shirt. The group worked on orders from outside organizations that needed the shirts for various functions. Each member of the team was paid a wage based on the ability to successfully complete the task and create a given number of T-shirts (based on what each patient could reasonably produce given her physical and cognitive limitations at that time). While at the print shop, Emily was able to learn how to focus on a specific task without being distracted by intrusive thoughts about how her life would never be the same again.

These activities helped Emily regain some of her executive functioning—for example, she might need to decide on a pattern for a specific vendor's job, and then remember the sequence of steps necessary to carry out the job. Furthermore, during the planning stages for each project, she and the group used their creativity to come up with novel prototypes from which the vendor could choose. In this environment, as well as in the auto shop, physical, occupational, and speech therapy occur in a "normal" setting through interesting activities. This approach circumvents the boredom of traditional therapy sessions that have little connection to the real world.

Leah Roberts, the victim of a stroke (from Chapter 6), was always happiest when it was her turn to cook in the group kitchen. Under the guidance of a rehabilitation specialist, she chopped vegetables, opened cans, and made an almost-from-scratch tomato sauce. In addition to relearning step-by-step sequential thinking and the social skills needed to set up a meal within the context of working in a group, she gave her muscles a great workout by expanding her range of motion as she reached for cabinet doors and strengthened her fine motor skills with every chop of the knife.

When she tried to teach a class for other residents in our program, Jessica Collins (whose accident is described in the Introduction) came to the sad realization that she couldn't ever return to being an aerobics teacher. She was able to see for herself how her disabilities would prevent her from actually being able to teach the exercises and lead a class. This was a far more powerful emotional learning experience for her than hearing about her limitations from the staff could ever have been. However, she also realized that she still wanted to remain physically fit, as this was very important to her self-image. To that end, she worked hard in the therapeutic gym with her physical and occupational therapists to develop routines that would produce the desired effects, while recognizing that she needed to learn new strategies to perform many of the activities that had come so naturally to her before the accident. When she returned home, she was able to continue to practice these strategies in her own home gym and attain her goal of remaining physically fit and in control of her weight.

THE GOALS OF POST-ACUTE REHABILITATION

Although post-acute rehabilitation cannot perform miracles and change biological realities, it can bridge the gap between acute hospital care and the return to home life, given the ever-shortening lengths of time that insurance companies allow for patients in hospital settings in today's economic environment. Post-acute rehabilitation facilities are designed to help ensure a successful transition from hospital to home by providing the needed continuity of care. This transition is critical to producing an optimal neurorehabilitation outcome following severe brain injury, especially for fragile patients with multiple disabilities. In these post-acute settings, the more home-like environment can serve as a model for what life will be like at home and give both the patient and his or her family a sense of the brain-injured person's capabilities. As a result, once the patient does return home, the family will be better prepared to accommodate the needs of its injured loved one.

TEAM PLAYERS

Like any successful venture, a rehabilitation center is only as good as its team. Some of the team players at a rehabilitation facility include the following professionals:

- *The medical director* is the team leader. This physician drives the treatment planning and medical and therapeutic strategies employed at each phase, much like a symphony conductor. She generally oversees and supervises the entire staff, working with the interdisciplinary team to establish a realistic treatment plan for each patient. This plan incorporates what she, through experience and wisdom, determines is medically probable, with important input from both the patient and his family. She is also responsible for managing medications, diagnosing medical disorders accompanying the injury and potential medical or neurobehavioral complications, and ensuring that the overall focus of a patient's therapeutic day reflects his treatment plan. Her specialty training may be in neurology, neuropsychiatry, or physical medicine and rehabilitation. A complete team usually has staff members from all three disciplines actively available (not just on a list of consultants) to help care for the patients on a regular basis.
- *Neuropsychologists* perform the psychological, behavioral, and neuropsychological testing, as well as cognitive therapies designed to help strengthen a patient's remaining abilities while compensating for deficits.
- *Clinical psychologists* provide counseling for patients and their families. This usually occurs in a teaching, cognitive-behavioral

manner (see Chapters 12 and 13) rather than through "talk therapy."

- *Physical therapists* provide help with lower-extremity motor functions, such as walking and navigating through different environments, including moving from a wheelchair to a car seat. They also help patients improve muscle tone, balance, and endurance.

- *Occupational therapists* help patients regain a whole host of skills. They are, in many ways, like "life coaches" in the rehabilitation world. Although their training is heavily weighted toward the treatment of upper-extremity and hand disabilities, they also help patients apply relearned abilities in everyday settings (such as during showering and dressing and in the performance of recreational activities).

- *Speech and language pathologists* help patients regain their ability to regulate speech and improve comprehension of language. They also work with reading comprehension, language expression, and some cognitive therapies. Another important role they play is to evaluate a patient's ability to swallow, helping to determine when a patient is no longer at risk of aspirating fluids or foods into the lungs, and deciding which dietary modifications are necessary for safe oral eating.

- *Rehabilitation nurses* are trained to administer medications and medical treatments, to educate patients on medication management, and to help patients with personal hygiene matters, including bladder and bowel management. Also, rehabilitation nurses participate in and reinforce lessons learned from therapy sessions, since they are available to the patient twenty-four hours a day, in contrast to rehabilitation treatment staff, who are usually on campus only during weekdays.

- *Social workers* spend much of their time working closely with the patient's family, providing support and compassion and fostering insight in individual sessions as well as group settings. They also assist with the practical implementation of the patient's treatment plan. For example, they may assist the patient and the family in determining how to obtain needed durable medical equipment and supplies necessary for the family to have at home prior to discharge.

- *Recreational therapists* work on the development of appropriate leisure activities. Many times, TBI patients are unable to relax and have fun in the same way they did prior to the injury. These therapists help patients identify new recreational pursuits or develop compensatory strategies to engage in their earlier interests.

- *Vocational therapists* help patients recognize their strengths and weaknesses in the workplace. They match the patient's strengths with work that is both available in the local community and interesting to the patient, and they improve the chances of success of an appropriate match by teaching patients how to rebuild their résumés, interview for a job, and work with potential employers. They also provide a liaison for both the patient and his supervisor to ease employment jitters. Finally, they may actually coach a patient at the workplace, helping him to overcome obstacles to completing work assignments, to organize his time effectively, to initiate additional work when appropriate, and to approach others in a respectful manner.

- *Art, music, and pet therapists* all encourage self-expression, helping patients discover new avenues of communication to help reduce stress. A pet therapist often brings animals on-site to provide companionship to those for whom the stress of multiple human interactions is overwhelming or who could benefit from learning to care for someone other than themselves.

- *Dieticians* work with the therapists and patients to ensure that daily nutritional needs are met while the patient is at the rehab center. They also help the patient prepare for the time when he will be on his own, teaching him how to plan his own meals and go shopping, or work with the family to prepare them for their loved one's special nutritional needs. When people become brain-injured, their nutritional needs may change. Some people lose a lot of weight during their early recovery. Others have a dysfunction in the area of the brain that controls hunger and may not know when to stop eating. Still others may need a special diet due to problems with swallowing.

- *Case managers* are the supportive liaisons between the patients and their funding sources—for example, insurance companies or governmental agencies. They keep an insurance carrier or governmental agency aware of a patient's ongoing needs so that the pressure to contain health-care costs doesn't occur at the expense of an individual's need for treatment. It is important to remember that it is the achievement of realistic goals that sets the time frame for treatment, not the number of days left on some bureaucrat's calendar. Ideally, the case manager remains involved with the patient and his family after discharge as well to monitor the patient's progress and the need for additional interventions if they arise.

All of these team members work closely together in an interdisciplinary format in which each specialist helps reinforce the skills learned in sessions with the other disciplines. For example, one therapist may help a patient relearn simple math skills, while another will build on these lessons to help him manage money. Yet another may reinforce the financial lessons by taking the patient to the bank and the mall. Throughout these activities, a patient's range of motion, balance, problem-solving capabilities, interactions with others, and other skills are used and strengthened, ultimately becoming part of a habit pattern for that activity. With practice, the ordinary activities that at first seem so difficult eventually require far less mental and physical work to perform. With this kind of interdisciplinary treatment, the TBI patient is in a better position to pursue new life goals after treatment ends and real life begins again.

In the next sections, we will review some some specific types of therapeutic interventions that are used in certain situations to help with rehabilitation and reduce handicaps. In the next chapter, we'll focus on some of the medication interventions that may benefit brain-injured individuals.

chapter 11

MEDICATION THERAPIES

> *They didn't give him medicine just to keep him*
> *quiet. They only gave him drugs that would*
> *help his aggression and anger at the lowest dose*
> *possible.*
>
> —Darrell Thorn, father of a young TBI
> patient

Bruce Robertson became delirious as he emerged from his coma. He began flailing about, screaming at the top of his lungs. He hallucinated about stethoscope snakes and monsters creeping out of the lights. He tugged and pulled at the IV lines that provided life-sustaining antibiotics. When it became clear that this was not just a brief, passing phase of his recovery, his doctor gave him a short-term course of intravenous haloperidol (Haldol) until the delirium passed.

Leah Roberts's right hand was curling up and looked a bit like a claw following the stroke to the left side of her brain. Her treatment team was concerned that her fingers might become so misshapen that they would permanently touch her palm. This sign of a condition called spasticity, common in the aftermath of TBI, made it difficult for Leah to perform daily activities. It was extremely painful. She was given an injection of botulinum, the generic name of Botox (the same drug that some dermatologists use for reducing facial wrinkles), directly into the contracted muscles, and gradually, with the aid of physical therapy and a splint, she was able to uncurl her hand.

Emily Carter was a cheerful person before her car accident, but her TBI left her depressed for months. For a time, she turned to street drugs, mainly cocaine, in an attempt to self-medicate. Her depression was stopping her from fully benefiting from rehabilitation. She also became unable to control her emotional outbursts, yelling at her mother and refusing to go to her outpatient therapy appointments. Fortunately, her depression lifted after she began taking an antidepressant, paroxetine (Paxil), and stopped using cocaine.

After Troy Atkins was admitted for post-acute rehabilitation several months after a bizarre gun accident caused a wound to his brain, I met with him to ensure that his medications were working in an optimal manner. He needed to adhere to his pharmaceutical regimen in order to be able to go back to school as soon as possible. He participated in many of the rehabilitation activities, but he did not need to relearn the activities of daily life. He currently takes Depakote to prevent possible seizures and help stabilize his mood, Zoloft for his depression, and Risperdal as needed to help during periods of disorganized thinking and irrational anger. The regimen is working: He's back at school.

As these examples show, psychopharmacology is less about the traumatic brain injury itself and more about secondary problems that occur in its aftermath.

Of course, in the immediate aftermath of a brain injury, medicine can save lives and keep a TBI from getting worse. But once the immediate crises have passed and a patient is either in post-acute rehabilitation or at home, secondary brain-based problems can become the foremost issues keeping the individual from reaching his or her full potential.

An Rx for Good Health

When it comes to traumatic brain injury, the medical mottos are "Less is more" and "Start low and go slow." Drugs should be correctly used to relieve symptoms and prevent further complications. Working with a single medication and administering the lowest possible dose will decrease the chances of undesirable side effects, which can include allergic reactions (such as itchy rashes), excess sleepiness, tremulousness, and nausea.

Drugs are not magic, but the careful use of pharmaceuticals can do wonders. Representing decades of intense research and scientific development, today's medicines can, in many cases, be used effectively to prevent chronic migraine headaches, improve spasticity, smooth erratic moods, and lift depression. They can also be used to prevent seizures and stop them when they do occur. They can help manage life-threatening delirium, which is a severe confusional state common in brain-injured patients, who may awake from a coma without being able to form new memories, recall old ones, or establish a normal sleep-wake cycle. This chapter will cover the medications most commonly used in brain-injury rehabilitation.

ANTIDEPRESSANTS

As we have seen, depression is extremely common in TBI patients, and sometimes it can interfere with rehabilitation: A depressed patient finds it hard to concentrate and listen, is not motivated, and may become suicidal. For these patients, the carefully supervised use of an antidepressant can help. Depression is currently believed to be caused by a number of factors, including genetic predisposition, environmental stressors, hormonal imbalances, and abnormal brain chemistry. Antidepressants work by helping to restore the proper balance of the neurotransmitters that are the basis for much of the brain's chemical activity.

Brain injury produces imbalances in these chemical messengers that disrupt their preinjury ebb and flow. After a brain injury, neuronal disruption makes it difficult for many individuals to appropriately respond to changes in their external environments and internal emotional states. These chemical abnormalities can often be corrected by the appropriate use of antidepressant medications.

Because brain injury may cause a heightened sensitivity to antidepressants and their potential side effects, lower-than-normal dosages can often be used to treat depression successfully and without significant adverse effects. However, patients must be watched for any unusual side effects, including suicidal thoughts, excessive drowsiness, and, paradoxically, mania, increased anxiety, and/or severe insomnia. The anxiety may be exacerbated by the fact that the patient is already under emotional stress because of the TBI, and the insomnia can have a big impact because the patient is probably already fatigued by the physical demands of rehabilitation.

Often, the antidepressants of choice are *selective serotonin reuptake inhibitors (SSRIs)*. Serotonin levels are usually lower in people who are depressed than in others. Serotonin is one of a group of neurotransmitters (*monoamines*) in the brain involved with mood. Under normal circumstances, it is released by a presynaptic neuron, crosses the fluid-filled synapse, and then interacts with specific receptors on the postsynaptic

WHO GETS DEPRESSED?

A study of over 650 TBI patients found that those most at risk for depression were unemployed and financially strapped. Younger people, students, and those soon to retire were less susceptible. Surprisingly, the severity of the injury and marital status were not significant risk factors. A person with severe TBI will rarely say that she is depressed—she will more likely demonstrate it by exhibiting the following symptoms: fatigue, inability to pay attention, and obsessive thinking.

neuron. If enough serotonin is released by the presynaptic neuron, the postsynaptic neuron will permit certain chemical changes to occur within this cell. These chemical changes will ultimately produce the electrical transmission of information, which occurs far more rapidly via electrical impulses than through chemical release. Once serotonin has produced its effects on the postsynaptic cell, remaining free molecules of serotonin may be recycled by being reabsorbed by the presynaptic neuron through a chemical "reuptake" mechanism so that it can be preserved to be used again. However, if the presynaptic cell does not require all of the remaining free serotonin, it is left within the synapse for degradation by enzymes that deactivate it, turning it into an inactive molecule. This process takes a longer time than reuptake, permitting the residual serotonin to continue to exert some effects on the postsynaptic neuron.

SSRI medications block serotonin from being recycled, thereby preventing its reuptake. In this way, more serotonin remains active within the synapse, which means it can have a greater effect on the postsynaptic neuron, enhancing its electrical transmission capability. Some of the SSRIs used for depressed TBI patients include fluoxetine (Prozac), paroxetine (Paxil), sertraline (Zoloft), escitalopram (Lexapro), and citalopram (Celexa).

Other types of antidepressants are not limited to blocking reuptake of serotonin. One class of these newer medications blocks the reuptake of norepinephrine, another monoamine neurotransmitter, as well as the reuptake of serotonin. These medications are called *selective serotonin and norepineph-rine reuptake inhibitors (SSNRIs)*. They include venlafaxine (Effexor) and mirtazapine (Remeron).

Other classes of antidepressant medications concentrate on inhibiting the reuptake of norepinephrine and dopamine. One example, bupropion (Wellbutrin), is often less sedating than some of the other antidepressants, but unlike the SSRIs and SSNRIs, it doesn't produce weight gain or sexual dysfunction (which are common side effects of SSRIs in both men and women).

Older classes of antidepressants—called *tricyclics*, based on their three-ring chemical structure—are still useful. They impact a whole array of neuro-transmitters, including all of the monoamines mentioned above, but have a different set of side effects, such as dry mouth, blurry vision, and constipa-tion. Three examples of this class of medications are impipramine (Tofranil), amitriptyline (Elavil), and nortriptyline (Pamelar). A review of fifty studies on antidepressants found that the *tricyclics* may give significant relief from the pain caused by damaged nerve tissue. They also are particu-larly helpful in preventing migraine headaches and improving emotional incontinence, a disorder in which a person frequently loses control of her emotions and can go from laughing to crying in just minutes.

BENZODIAZEPINES (BDZ) TO REDUCE ANXIETY AND PROMOTE SLEEP

Antianxiety drugs called *benzodiazepines (BDZ)* are usually used for short-term management of debilitating anxiety or insomnia; they can also help reduce the pain of muscle spasms in TBI patients. Like the antidepressants, they must be closely monitored. Side effects may include disinhibition, am-nesia, excess drowsiness, and possible dependence on their use. Once the underlying condition that produced the insomnia has been resolved through the use of a more specific medication and/or therapy, the benzodi-azepine should be discontinued, as it can be addictive with long-term use. Insomnia is a common symptom of depression, for example, and should resolve once the underlying depression is appropriately treated. The danger

MEMORY LOST AND FOUND

Research suggests that a medication already used to treat Alzheimer's disease may help moderate to severe TBI patients with memory loss. Called rivastigmine (Exelon), it works by increasing the neurotransmitter acetylcholine, which is responsible for many memory and learning capabilities. A 2006 study found that 30 percent of moderate to severely brain-injured patients taking rivastigmine remembered more words and paid better attention to given tasks when compared to TBI patients who were not given the drug.

A newer class of medications currently used for the management of primary dementia, including memantine (Namenda), principally work by blocking the flow of ions through channels of N-methyl-d-aspartate (NMDA) receptors—a glutamate (chemically an amino acid) receptor subfamily broadly involved in brain function and present on certain neurons. Memantine has been tried with some success in brain injury survivors to help improve their memory deficits. Like all medications, these drugs have side effects that may limit their use.

In a twist of irony, people with TBI **may be at increased risk of dementia, or may begin to suffer from it at an earlier age,** especially if they have had other family members diagnosed with it. In one study, TBI patients under age seventy-five were found to be twice as likely as their noninjured peers to develop Alzheimer's. This may be a reason to consider using these groups of medications earlier in the management of memory problems that are caused by brain injury.

is that a patient in the early stages of addiction may increase his or her dose without medical supervision. Some BDZs include alprazolam (Xanax), chlordiazepoxide (Librium), clonazepam (Klonopin), diazepam (Valium), and lorazepam (Ativan).

ANTIPSYCHOTICS TO HELP ORGANIZE THINKING

Antipsychotic drugs help manage disorganized thinking and delirium and reduce irrational or unwanted thoughts and hallucinations. It is not entirely clear what causes psychotic symptoms in patients with TBI (or in other psychotic patients), but again the monoamine neurotransmitters seem to play a role. Loss of contact with the real world and an inability to perceive things clearly can create unpredictable and destructive behavior.

Antipsychotics are now classified into two groups, based on both their neurotransmitter effects and the side effects most commonly seen in them. The first group, encompassing many of the older antipsychotics, such as haloperidol (Haldol), chlorpromazine (Thorazine), and thioridazine (Mellaril), can successfully treat the symptoms of psychosis. However, in approximately 20 percent of patients treated with these medications, an often irreversible neurological side effect known as *tardive dyskinesia* develops, thus limiting their use in recent years. Tardive dyskinesia produces abnormal involuntary motor movements in many parts of the body, especially in the tongue and lips (uncontrollable lip-smacking being one example). The newer antipsychotics—often referred to as second-generation, or atypical, antipsychotics—do not produce this problem and are now the drugs of choice for management of psychotic symptoms, except for delirium. Examples of these drugs are risperidone (Risperdal), olanzapine (Zyprexa), and quetiapine (Seroquel). But they are not free of side effects, which include diabetes and weight gain.

The atypical antipsychotic medication clozapine (Clozaril), discovered in the 1960s, was not allowed to be used in the United States until 1989 due to side effects associated with unacceptably low white-blood-cell counts. Since then, its use has remained under strict guidelines. Clozapine remains the gold standard for all antipsychotics, however, because of its effectiveness in patients who don't respond to any of the other available medications. Interestingly, instead of producing tardive dyskinesia, this medication actually improves it.

Norepinephrine Blockers to Stop Anxiety and Uncontrollable Anger

Norepinephrine blockers can work in both the peripheral and the central nervous systems, literally blocking the anxiety-creating neurotransmitters that instruct the body to raise blood pressure, increase heart rate, and begin sweating and shaking, all while pounding home a migraine headache. These agents may help TBI patients who have uncontrollable anger and aggression by reducing the bodily sensations that can worsen an already bad situation. Some of these medications also stop tremors, without producing drowsiness, making them useful in certain anxiety-provoking situations because they leave the person with a clearer head. Patients taking these medications must be carefully monitored to ensure that their blood pressure does not drop too low.

ANTICONVULSANTS, OR ANTIEPILEPTIC DRUGS, TO STOP SEIZURES AND STABILIZE MOOD

Anticonvulsants, also called *antiepileptic drugs (AED),* both stop and prevent the convulsions, or seizures, that affect many brain-injured patients. They may also soothe aggression and stabilize the emotions of patients prone to mood swings. At one time, it was de rigueur to give all TBI patients anticonvulsants, but today their use varies. In some centers, they are now given only if there is a second witnessed seizure; in others they are still seen as the standard of care. (However, recent studies show that giving the AED phenytoin as a prophylactic measure to patients with severe TBI in the early stages of recovery can prevent posttraumatic seizures—during the first week only.)

Older anticonvulsants, such as phenobarbital, cause sedation and cognition problems and are reserved only for inducing a coma, which is sometimes required for patients with severe TBIs. Many Level I Neurotrauma Centers continue to prefer to administer medications that may prevent seizures to severely brain-injured patients once they reach the emergency room. Because these patients are in coma, they cannot be given oral medications to ward off potential seizures; therefore an older anticonvulsant, phenytoin (Dilantin), remains in use, as it can be readily administered intravenously.

Following acute neurotrauma care, most physicians who follow these patients during their neurorehabilitation use newer generations of anticonvulsants, including carbamazepine (Tegretol), oxcarbazepine (Trileptal), valproate (Depakene or Depakote), or lamotrigine (Lamictal), which have fewer long-term cognitive side effects than phenytoin.

Lithium Carbonate to Balance Moods

Long the drug of choice for mood swings, lithium carbonate is a natural salt. It quiets the raging range of moods that many brain-injured patients feel and stabilizes their lives. It is a medication that must be monitored by blood levels, as levels that are too high can produce cardiac and central nervous system toxicity. Some other possible side effects are increased urination, tremors, confusion, and hypothyroidism.

Stimulants to Reduce Distraction and Impulsivity

The same psychostimulants that are given to hyperactive children can also help some brain-injured patients who have problems concentrating and show signs of impulsiveness or hyperactivity. They are also used when a TBI patient is sleepy and lethargic during the day. Many of these medications increase the amount of the neurotransmitter dopamine, which when deficient prevents the frontal lobes from exercising their executive functions. Some psychostimulants are methylphenidate (Ritalin), amphetamine (Dexedrine), and pemoline (Cylert). A 2004 study of the effects of methylphenidate on patients with TBI found that it significantly improved their speed of processing information and ability to pay attention.

Although not a stimulant, modafinil (Provigil) is a new drug that induces wakefulness, in part by its action in the anterior *hypothalamus* and the reticular activating system. Unlike the stimulants, it does not become habit-forming, increase heart rate or blood pressure, or produce the other side effects seen with traditional stimulants. Studies have shown that this medication may improve alertness during both the early and late phases of recovery.

Because all of these medications need to be closely supervised, initiating pharmacotherapy often works best within the safe environment of a hospital or post-acute rehabilitation facility. Keep in mind that in TBI patients, drugs are more likely to produce side effects even at low doses. A physician should not prescribe any medication until a detailed medical history has been taken and a complete neurological examination completed.

Thought. Perception. Memory. These and other areas of cognition can be damaged by TBI, and they need more than medication to be helped. In the next section, you will learn how rehabilitation can help with the loss of cognitive powers.

chapter 12

COGNITIVE THERAPY

Set your goals, work hard, and trust the people out there who are helping you.

—Ricky Parker, father, husband, and TBI survivor

When Jessica Collins first came to her rehabilitation facility, she was severely brain-injured. She could breathe on her own and swallow, but that was about all. One of the first things her occupational therapist taught her was how to regain management of her bladder and bowel routines. Jessica learned to use a timer that she kept clipped to her wheelchair, which buzzed every two hours as a "cue" to go to the bathroom before an embarrassing crisis developed.

Y. J. Ming has come a long way since he was first admitted for early rehabilitation after his heart attack. Now that he is at home, however, he still forgets to do certain tasks—or how to do them once he starts. He needs help remembering to make his own lunch, for example, and how to choose foods that will help keep his heart healthy. But he has learned over a number of years how to compensate for these memory deficits and uses various strategies routinely to accomplish "must-do" things. The first step was to develop a "cueing mechanism" that didn't rely on his memory to let him know when it was time to eat or carry out other essential tasks. Like many other brain-injury survivors, he could not remember to check the time when he was busy doing other things. The prolonged loss of oxygen to his brain that occurred as a result of his sudden heart attack produced damage that just could not be repaired.

The solution was to set the alarm on his watch to go off at various times during the day. The alarm cues him to check a notebook that contains his daily schedule. Then he matches the time on his watch with the activity associated with it on his schedule and shifts his focus to attending to it. So, if it is lunchtime, he goes into the kitchen, where a large whiteboard on the wall lists each step he needs to perform to make his lunch. He has also learned that it is best if he reads each step out loud to make sure he gets it right. As an example, the steps might start out like this:

1. Wash your hands.
2. Open the refrigerator.
3. Remove the bread from the refrigerator.
4. Remove the butter from the refrigerator.
5. Put bread and butter on kitchen table.

And so on. Otherwise, he might forget a step and require his wife's help to prepare a simple meal. Practical solutions like this make a huge difference in his marriage. His wife doesn't have to plan her day around Y.J.'s needs, which permits her to volunteer at the school their child attends and still have time that is hers alone. Without that time off, she would be at risk of burning out.

John Lewis was lucky that his brain injury was "mild." Even so, his cognitive deficits meant he just couldn't go back to his detail-oriented, fast-paced life as an insurance salesman. In order to be able to work three days a week at the real estate information service run by his wife, Gloria, he had to learn how to use a computer all over again. However, he found he was unable to multitask; he had trouble with some of his assignments (such as making copies and collating the pages); and he couldn't remember the delivery route he was required to run to take information to vendors. Given how important this job was to his self-esteem, we established a plan in cognitive therapy sessions that would enable John to succeed.

Gloria now makes a list of his assignments and allows John lots of time to complete each step along the way. He begins his day much earlier than before and follows the outline that Gloria has prepared, whether he agrees with it or not. The printing jobs that used to confuse him are done by another assistant, and John is in charge of stapling together the finished product. As time went by, Gloria learned that her customers really enjoyed the time that John spent with them each day—he often delivered coffee and donuts to the offices along with the booklets, things that Gloria never had time to do when she was running the operation on her own—so John knows that he is making a valuable contribution to the business doing something he is good at.

A big life adjustment for the both of them? Yes, but life has now assumed some normalcy and John feels productive once again. This is truly what successful rehabilitation is all about. Despite everything, they both now have a quality of life that actually surpasses the one they had before John's accident.

Cognitive therapy is a comprehensive, multipronged method of retraining brain-injured people to carry out the tasks of everyday life so they can be as independent as possible. These tasks include such basics as going to the bathroom unaided as well as more complicated activities, such as balancing a checkbook or collating the pages of a printout. As we have seen, brain injuries often result in damage to the areas of the brain most responsible for focusing attention, planning and sequencing tasks, remembering new things, making sound judgments, and having self-awareness. Helping brain-injured people regain the ability to carry out these basic thought processes is one of the greatest challenges of rehabilitation.

Depending on the location of the brain injury, the mechanism of injury, and the severity of injury, certain cognitive capabilities may slowly return over time, especially if coupled with appropriate help from experienced professionals. These specially trained therapists work with patients on retraining parts of the brain and teach compensatory strategies for areas that are not yet capable of being retrained. They also help patients with severe TBIs accept some of the cognitive deficits that may *not* be responsive to either retraining or compensation. Often, such limitations are based on the number and severity of the residual lesions that, for example, may make understanding oral or written communication impossible, thereby limiting the options available for compensation.

Areas that the interdisciplinary team addresses in patients with cognitive deficits are usually organized to deal with the disabilities that are initially the most handicapping to the individual. Disabilities that prevent the individual from performing skills required to manage his most basic personal needs usually take the highest priority. These are the areas that are the greatest barriers to returning to some form of independence. They may include:

- Personal hygiene
- Consistency in following a daily routine
- Social skills necessary to form relationships
- Appropriate interpersonal interactions, such as maintaining an appropriate distance from other people and therefore not making them uncomfortable by "violating their personal space"
- Memory
- Relearning ways to ensure safety

Interdisciplinary rehab team members work together closely to reach these goals, incorporating basic tenets of cognitive therapy into their respective therapeutic interventions with the patient. In addition to more general activities, each patient is seen by therapists for sessions that focus on helping him perform specific cognitive tasks. These sessions are individualized to maximize the benefit for the patient as he practices tasks. The activities themselves are based on the patient's abilities and designed to overcome specific deficits.

In the treatment environment, cognitive therapy includes all therapeutic interactions with staff members that involve problem-solving skills. As an example, let's say a patient becomes frustrated when trying to rewrite her résumé as part of an assignment for a job reentry class, and she storms out of the computer lab and into her room. Her assigned staff member follows her to her room but, before approaching her, allows her a few minutes to cool down (as long as the patient's frustration does not place her or others at risk of harm). Immediate interaction tends to worsen the individual's frustration by introducing social pressure for her to respond to another person while in the midst of an intense personal reaction to the precipitating event.

After several minutes, the therapist asks the patient if she would like "some coaching." If she agrees, the therapist may begin the coaching conversation by asking the patient, "Did storming out of the lab help you accomplish your goal?" It is never helpful for the therapist to assume that he fully understands the rationale for the patient's current problem. Any number of hypothetical reasons for the expression of frustration may be imagined—such as computer malfunction, fatigue, intrusive thoughts, or annoyance at another individual. However, for this to be a helpful intervention, the patient's reasons for the breakdown must be fully explored and each major issue written down. Part of the therapeutic interaction is having the patient find a way to express her rationale for the breakdown, so that the therapist can evaluate it in the context of the current environment.

As discussed in Chapter 6, perception and reasoning are important aspects of cognition. In this example, the patient's perception may have been distorted by her inability to focus her eyes on the small text on the screen (resulting from a deficit in eyesight known as *convergence* that is a symptom of most TBIs). Her misunderstanding of the reason for this difficulty may have led her to think that she could never learn how to use a computer again. The staff intervention involves not only teaching the patient how to adjust the size of the fonts in the word-processing program, but also helping her realize that her reaction reflected a number of errors in reasoning based on her faulty perception. Finally, the therapist would help her explore alternative ways of thinking about the situation that could allow her to avoid exploding in similar frustrating situations in the future.

BREAKING DOWN TASKS INTO STEPS

Teaching brain-injured people is not like what a history teacher does when teaching her students. A teacher typically gives tests to students to see how much of the material presented in her lectures actually got incorporated into the students' store of new knowledge. This type of learning by the students, called *declarative learning,* which involves listening to the instructor's words, taking notes, asking questions, and remembering the information presented in the class, requires a fully intact central nervous system. But learning is mediated by memory, and there are many areas of the brain involved in memory and learning.

Learning in fact is predicated on both short- and long-term memory. Short-term memory can be so impaired by deficits in attention and concentration that new learning cannot take place; facts and new information cannot be remembered even briefly. Under such circumstances, there is no possibility of new learning being incorporated into long-term memory.

Long-term memory has two major subdivisions, explicit and implicit memory. *Explicit memory* generally involves the use of language; when used in the context of learning it is associated with the kind of *declarative learning* that the history teacher is concerned with. *Implicit memory,* in contrast, does not require the use of conscious thought. When implicit memory is used in learning, it is called *procedural learning* or *motor learning.* This is the kind of learning that permits us to learn how to ride a bicycle, play the piano, or dance. When procedural learning occurs, prior experience and practice permit us to perform tasks such as brushing our teeth without conscious attention. In daily life, we rely on procedural learning that is retained as implicit memory to perform a variety of routine tasks, permitting us to focus on other matters that require problem-solving through the use of conscious processes.

For example, in the morning while making breakfast for the family, many people are capable of talking on the phone or discussing the day with a spouse. They might plan their work schedules or discuss complex scheduling problems while scrambling eggs and making coffee. Recent research into implicit memory and procedural learning has discovered why:

Carrying out a task like making breakfast—which is the result of implicit memory—uses completely different neuronal pathways than those employed to discuss the day, which are the result of short-term, or working, memory and declarative learning. Following a severe injury to the brain, patients can often relearn tasks, but it takes practice and it must call upon special strategies of using implicit memory and conditioned learning.

Through procedural learning, a severely brain-injured patient can become adept at finding his way to his room at the rehab center, even if he does not retain the ability to understand the kind of instructions that would normally be given (such as "Go down the hallway and turn left, then a quick right, and take the third door on the right"). Furthermore, if he was asked, "How do you get to your room?" he would find the question nonsensical and just shrug his shoulders.

Other types of cognitive therapy involve breaking down a task that a patient needs to relearn into its essential, component steps using language to facilitate its communication. (Y. J. Ming's list for preparing his lunch is a good example.) Each step is a lesson in problem-solving, organizing, remembering, and sequencing. Each step is linked to the next in a chain of actions that ultimately come together to complete a task.

A patient learns by going over and over the basic motor tasks that he once did without even thinking about them. But now he does have to think about them, and breaking down tasks into steps is very helpful, especially early on in the rehabilitation process when a patient has serious deficits in self-control, the ability to read, and the ability to follow a schedule.

Here is an example of a chain of commands, often referred to as a *chaining hierarchy,* utilized to help an individual get dressed after bathing:

1. Walk to dresser.
2. Open top dresser drawer, labeled "underwear and socks."
3. Remove undershirt (or bra) from the top drawer.
4. Remove underpants from the top drawer.
5. Remove socks from the top drawer.
6. Close the drawer.
7. Walk over to the bed, carrying the underwear and socks.
8. Put the underpants, undershirt (or bra), and socks on the bed.

9. Walk back to the dresser.
10. Open second dresser drawer, labeled "shirts."
11. Remove one shirt from the second drawer.
12. Close the drawer.
13. Walk over to the bed, carrying the shirt.
14. Put the shirt on the bed.
15. Walk back to the dresser.
16. Open third dresser drawer, labeled "pants."
17. Walk over to the bed, carrying the pants.

The list may go on to include many more steps, with each step clearly defined in the minutest detail. At the early stage of treatment, staff members read the lists out loud to the patient and help her physically complete each step, even if that requires hands-on personal assistance. Depending on the needs of the individual patient and her capacity for learning, this routine may be done several times each day rather than just once in the morning. Unfortunately, this amount of repetition is often overlooked in generic rehab programs that are not focused on the most important things a patient must learn before he is ready for less supervised care.

In time, if the steps a patient uses to get dressed are repeated over and over again in the same order, they will become part of the brain-injured patient's implicit memory. This happens as the declarative learning that occurs through the use of "cues" comes to feel like part of an automatic routine via procedural learning. Once procedural learning has occurred, the patient will be able to get dressed completely on his own or perhaps need only some intermittent cueing from the staff or his family. Once a routine is reestablished, it becomes far easier for a brain-injured individual to perform because it does not require new learning and relies only on unconscious (procedural) learning stored in implicit memory.

THE PERSONAL JOURNAL

Despite the many techniques and treatments available today, even the best therapist and the most motivated patient can only do so much. Repetition, chaining of commands, cueing—all these can help—but the injured brain can go only so far. Some tasks are just beyond a person's capacity because of the nature of the damage. Furthermore, rehabilitation progress moves slowly; there needs to be some sort of compensatory strategy to follow until the abilities that can come back do come back.

This is where a personal journal—called a *memory book* at many centers—comes into play. This is one of the most important tools a patient has to help her lead an independent life. The journal provides a single, organized source where explicit memory can be centralized using verbal learning. Further, it anticipates specific scenarios that may affect a patient's safety and uses written instructions, stated in understandable terms and ordered in a step-by-step fashion, that she can follow if and when such situations present themselves.

A personal journal contains everything from daily schedules to well-established "chaining hierarchies," or sequences of steps needed to accomplish various basic tasks. The journal should also contain current personal information, such as the name of the rehab center and its phone number; the patient's room number, Social Security number, and insurance information; the patient's important personal information, such as home address, phone number, date of birth, and the names of loved ones, nurses, therapists, and physicians; and important addresses and telephone numbers, including a boldly written single-page message: "When in danger, call 911." In sum, the journal contains all the things a patient must be able to quickly access to ensure safety and become as independent as possible.

I purposely use the term "personal journal" rather than the more standard "memory book" because the latter tends to remind an individual that he is "damaged," and this constant reminder can be an impediment to keeping a journal. Also, unlike a "memory book," a personal journal is so much more than just a memory aid. It is a way for an individual to express feelings, recall things she wishes to discuss with her doctor, remind herself of the progress she has made in therapy, and reconnect her past with her current life, however different it may be.

This personal journal becomes central to the rehabilitation of patients who can utilize explicit memory and language to compensate for memory deficits that cannot be cured. The patients who are able to embrace using a personal journal as part of their new lives, not as just another externally imposed therapeutic task, have far better outcomes in being able to maximize independence than those who choose to see it as something that can be discarded upon returning home.

CREATING THE RIGHT ENVIRONMENT

A brain-injured person's cognitive abilities and limitations require an environment that compensates for these limitations yet allows the patient to employ his strengths to enhance learning and reduce stress. Most hospital treatment environments are designed for rapid patient turnover and contain a plethora of medical gadgets, many of which beep and squeal whenever an alarm goes off. Of course, such intensive monitoring is necessary in acute situations, but, for neurologic patients, this noise and confusion causes undue stress for an already overwhelmed and injured brain. The brain is not accurately processing the information spewing forth in this environment, and this causes anxiety to set in, which leads to more confusion. The stress associated with being in a hospital and feeling out of control is very frustrating for an already short-fused person with a brain injury. Such conditions can easily elicit the expression of understandable but dysfunctional behavior, such as impulsiveness and aggression. Furthermore, all of this external confusion worsens the patient's internal confusion, which makes learning nearly impossible.

It is important for therapists to get to know each patient as an individual and figure out how to modify the environment so that frustrations and distractions are minimized and learning can take place. For example, some patients require frequent breaks during treatment sessions, a time to retreat to the solitude of their rooms, close the door, dim the lights, and escape the din of the more public rooms. Some patients, when asked about their feelings of anxiety, are able to calm themselves and even identify the particular cause of the stress reaction. If so, the therapist should encourage this, however trivial the cause of the anxiety may sound, allowing the patient to give voice to the feelings that were invoked. The point is to identify the causes of distress and then make changes in the environment to counter them and provide a milieu where a patient can be successfully rehabilitated.

THE ISSUE OF SELF-AWARENESS

Without at least some self-awareness on the part of the patient, rehabilitation can be a real challenge. Lack of self-awareness occurs with anosognosia (see Chapter 7). People cannot learn unless they are aware of what they are doing—and why they are doing it. One of the most important and challenging areas of cognitive remediation involves reestablishing self-awareness—helping the patient understand that he has had a brain injury and that he has certain disabilities, but that they need not create lasting handicaps that preclude a productive and fulfilling life.

A 2003 study showed that TBI patients with self-awareness were better able to perform the activities of daily living. That same study found that patients who regained only very minimal insight were more apt to minimize their deficits; they were not grounded in reality, and they thought they were able to do more than their therapists and caregivers knew they could. This situation can become problematic when, for example, an anosognosic TBI survivor with short-term memory loss insists on doing something dangerous, such as driving a car.

One of my patients, a former stockbroker, for example, understands that he had an injury, and after eight years he is able to live a relatively normal life with his wife and children. However, he continues to experience one big problem—because of his diminished self-awareness and impaired capacity for self-reflection about his own behavior, he remains unable to accept that he is no longer the head of his household. He believes he should be able to drive a car whenever he wishes, when in reality his judgment is so impaired that he just cannot do it safely. Unable to recognize the change in his circumstances, he inappropriately blames the most supportive person in his life—his wife—for trying to control him and "keep him under her thumb."

Teaching self-awareness is easier said than done. Traditional one-on-one therapy is not likely to work with a brain-injured individual with anosognosia. Because the patient has lost the ability to be self-reflective, she can't easily recognize which behaviors need to change and what options for changes exist within her current constraints. In addition, because of her short-term memory deficits, a traditional talk therapist can't ask her to delve into the roots of her chronic discontent; she may be unable to remember the most important parts of her previous sessions. Instead, a therapist must use what is called *paradigmatically oriented, modified cognitive behavioral therapy,* a basic nonreflective therapy that I have used successfully for over twenty-five years.

In this type of therapy, I sit with my TBI patient and explain, point-blank, what I see and my thoughts on what has to change if the patient wants to achieve the goals that he has set for himself. I actively point out inconsistencies in his thinking and encourage him to learn "scripts" that, when committed to memory via repetition, will enable him to respond to a general set of common life issues with greater success. When he is able to use these scripts in his own life and begins to receive positive feedback from those who are present in his world, he can see the success of this approach for himself and begins to utilize it with less and less prompting.

Although those of us who work in the field of neurorehabilitation can easily describe the types of cognitive deficits that a patient shows in rehabilitation settings, this information, when provided by therapy staff, is never as powerful as the feedback given to the patient by the real world. Thus, feedback from family, friends, and peers is far more effective than insights from therapists in helping a patient see that his issues and problems are not just confined to the rehabilitation setting.

Another valuable tool used in cognitive therapy is video-recording of both individual and group therapy sessions. The recordings are reviewed by both therapist and patient so that there is no mistaking the actions that actually occurred during sessions. Although there may be disagreements about why a particular event occurred, the recording permits them to analyze the event in detail and discuss alternative explanations for what occurred, as well as different ways that the situation could have been handled by the patient.

Family and friends are vital for reestablishing the individual's sense of self. I rely on information from them to help round out the experiences that my patients have written about in their journals, ensuring that there is some relationship between a real event and the one recorded in the patient's journal. I use their feedback to help my patients begin to understand that their own perceptions of themselves may not jibe with what others see about them. Patiently, over and over again, I attempt to explain interactions between the patient and other people with an attempt at broadening the patient's acceptance of differing points of view. I encourage family members and friends to reinforce the therapy sessions with the same one-on-one techniques at home.

Paradigmatically oriented therapy takes a long time. A trusting, involved, and supportive relationship between patient and therapist does not occur overnight, and neither does the process of gradually reawakening a brain-injured person's self-awareness. There is no epiphany, no "Eureka! I got it!" Instead, there is a very gradual understanding on the part of the patient that she is different following the injury and that others may well perceive her as different. Then, and only then, will the journey toward acceptance of this new self begin.

Above all, with these cognitive therapy techniques and others, a therapist must be patient—and he must instill that patience into the brain-injured person and his family. We all want results immediately in this fast-paced world, but in the realm of brain injury, progress is measured over many weeks or months, not session by session.

Ultimately, therapies directed at improving cognition are also designed to impact a person's behavior, the observable manifestations of thought. The next chapter takes these therapeutic techniques a step further, introducing behavioral therapy strategies that are helpful for brain-injured individuals. Behavioral therapy is a powerful tool in shaping human behavior; therefore, it is extremely important that such therapeutic strategies are well thought out, individualized, and consistently enforced as they are incorporated into the individual's interdisciplinary treatment plan.

chapter 13

BEHAVIORAL THERAPY

> *Those with great character always seem to survive.*
>
> —Paul, father, grandfather, husband, and TBI survivor

Sixteen-year-old Troy Atkins was easygoing, had lots of friends, and did well in school. His passion was skeet shooting. He clearly had Olympic potential and was preparing for the day when he could represent his country on the athletic battlefield. Then, one day, his whole life changed. He went skeet shooting with his dad, and the barrel of a malfunctioning rifle hurtled backward, becoming embedded in his brain. Luckily, Troy survived, but he was severely brain injured.

The result was a whole host of problems at home and especially at school. Although he continued to experience short-term memory deficits and executive dysfunction, his native intelligence was often able to cover for these problems. However, Troy's personality changed. He became belligerent. He yelled at his high-school teachers and hit two classmates. His anger soon turned to fear and anxiety—so much so that he couldn't stand being alone. Eventually, nearly three years after his original injury, after exhausting all local resources, his doctor asked me to see Troy and his family.

First, we collected every shred of information about what had happened to his brain, both at the time of the accident and during those crucial weeks following it. Then, we began forming a treatment plan. Because I elected to change a number of the medications Troy was on, his family and I felt that admission to our post-acute residential center was the safest way to proceed in implementing these changes. Part of the problem with his preadmission regimen appeared to be that he was on too many medications that fell into too many classes. I thought that the medications could be working at cross purposes. Our goal was to produce a new pharmacological plan that would help to balance out Troy's behavior. Medications can help an individual get "back in the ball game," but they were never designed to actually hit the balls that are pitched to him in the real game of life.

Troy quickly improved while living at the center and receiving appropriate therapy. He was able to return home and then finish high school. At that point, he wanted to go to college. His family and I felt that his condition was stable enough that he was ready to give it a try. He enrolled in a nearby community college and decided to commute from home rather than live in a dormitory with all its associated distractions. But some situations, usually new ones that came at him out of the blue, could still put him over the edge. Although Troy was no longer as anxious or angry as he was when we first met, he was still easily flustered when a teacher gave him a new assignment. In subsequent outpatient consultations, I worked with him and his mother to develop some strategies, in a loosely designed behavioral program, to help him deal with these situations.

First, I suggested that he ask his instructors to e-mail any new assignments to him on his Blackberry. We prepared a highly structured study plan that required him to devote sufficient time to his work each day (usually three hours) rather than attempting to cram before a test. We worked on reorganizing his bedroom to minimize distractions and established routines that would not require him to think about where he had put things he needed to find. For example, he bought a wall-mounted key holder that he labeled for each set of keys; the very first thing he would do when he entered his room was to hang his keys on the labeled hook (a suggestion that

I myself have followed for years). That way, he did not have to rely on short-term memory to remember where he had put them.

When a brain is injured, both its neurochemistry and its electrical activity are disrupted, although not always permanently, as we have seen in examples of mild cases of TBI (see Appendix A for more on neurotransmitters). Some of these neurotransmitters are designed to inhibit actions. Damage to their modulating influences often leads to *disinhibition,* permitting basic emotional drive states to be expressed in inappropriate personal or social situations. In other words, if a person with a brain injury feels something, regardless of what it may be, he is likely to blurt it out or act on it, unscreened by the brain's executive functions. As you can imagine from personal experience, especially when you may have had too much to drink, this kind of impulsivity can be very hurtful to others, as well as to yourself. Manners and civility go out the window when impulsivity and chaos rule.

In fact, the traits we usually associate with bad behavior—the outbursts, the violence, the impulse actions—can, for the most part, *result* from an inability to solve problems caused by the disruption of certain neurotransmitter systems in the brain. In order for a brain-injured individual to become a functioning member of society, he must relearn how to engage in the consistent, appropriate behavior that is necessary to successfully live and work with others.

We humans evolved to be a social species, and that means that our collective survival is dependent upon the ability to band together as functional groups and accomplish what no single individual could do by himself. Thus, if a person doesn't act appropriately, he can lose his family, his friends, and his job; he can risk the vital support so necessary for his recovery and reentry into the world. To be truly independent, a TBI patient must learn how to act with social appropriateness—and that's often where behavioral therapy comes in.

Before appropriate behavior can be taught, floridly inappropriate behavior must be brought under control. Aggression, violence, promiscuity—these first must be addressed. Consistent behavioral interventions incorporated into the team's treatment plan for the patient, often coupled with psychopharmacology, are usually successful in addressing maladaptive behavior. However, poorly thought out or incompletely executed behavior therapy can be worse than none at all. Its implementation is not to be taken lightly.

How It Works

Behavioral therapy works on the basis of two simple strategies: rewarding the good and ignoring the bad. First, a patient is rewarded or reinforced when appropriate behavior is actually demonstrated. To understand this behavioral strategy, think about this quote from the classic book *One-Minute Manager*: "Catch someone doing it right." For example, our rehab team is always on the lookout for spontaneous acts of kindness that one resident will offer to another or to a staff member. When this occurs, the resident offering the assistance is given a thank-you note that describes the exact nature of his act and the impact that the gesture had upon the other person. These cards are read with the resident and then the resident usually pins the card to the corkboard in his room. For less-impaired patients, this attention and praise is a positive social reward.

For a more impaired patient, for whom words and praise don't mean that much, a tangible reward swiftly following the expression of appropriate behavior must be employed. This person might get a favorite food or a drink of soda after showing just five minutes of controlled behavior. In this patient group, the frequency and rapid pairing of a consumable reward—food or drink—following the desired behavior is essential to condition the patient to associate the reward with the expressed behavior.

The next step is substituting some type of token, rather than immediate munchies, for demonstrating the desired behavior. This type of behavioral programming is one that airlines have successfully employed with all of us for years—frequent-flyer membership reward programs. Just as we travelers accumulate miles (tokens) that we can use toward "free" travel, patients accumulate points that can be exchanged for something they want that is not usually available to everyone at the center. These tangible rewards might include watching an extra hour of TV, having special one-on-one time with a favorite staff member, or going on an outing to a place of the patient's choice when the patient accumulates a given number of those valuable "frequent great behavior" points. These rewards reinforce, or more technically speaking, increase the frequency of, a desired behavioral response that will help a person regain internal control of her own life.

The second basic behavioral strategy is to ignore bad behavior. As simple as this sounds, the adage "the squeaky wheel gets the grease" is as much in evidence in some untrained staff approaches to patient management as it is in the real world. We humans are wired such that we crave attention, even if it's negative attention. We'd rather argue and fight than be ignored. Kids racing down the hallway at night love to have their parents scream at them to get back into bed. They want a reaction. So what happens if parents just ignore the attention-seeking behavior instead of reacting? Both theory and experience demonstrate that ignoring the behavior will lead to its rapid extinction (going away), as it just doesn't get the desired response anymore. There's no fun in the game if the parents don't start screaming and begin the chase down the hallway.

In rehabilitation, most aggressive behavior that is not harmful to the patient or to others is not criticized. Instead, it's ignored and a reward isn't given out.

Here's an example of behavioral training in a therapeutic setting using the above principles:

1. The usually loud and interruptive TBI patient is quiet for fifteen minutes while a therapist begins a discussion of current events.
2. He is given a token (for example, a gold star, or a check mark on a tabulation sheet) to start accumulating those great behavior points and praised by the therapist or another staff member.
3. He continues to be quiet, listening to the therapist for another fifteen minutes.
4. He is given another gold star as the therapist or other staff member again praises him, clearly pairing the star with the expression of the desired behavior.

5.   The more fifteen-minute periods of controlled behavior, the more gold stars. The more gold stars, the more privileges and rewards.

6.   Forty-five minutes into the class, the patient interrupts the therapist and starts yelling, "I want to leave!" "I want to leave now!"

7.   Rather than being punished or losing points (technically called a cost response), he is ignored. He just doesn't earn a gold star or points toward a reward. Nor does he get the attention he wanted from his outburst.

8.   He stops yelling. Fifteen minutes later, after once again demonstrating appropriate behavior, he earns another coveted gold star.

9.   In short, appropriate behavior is rewarded and inappropriate behavior is ignored.

10. The result? Appropriate behavior is gradually shaped and becomes routinized.

Jessica Collins, the former aerobics instructor, had always been a strong-willed person; she could stand up to the best and never feel sorry for herself. But after her severe TBI, things changed. She cried all the time. She'd shout at her mother, Laura, "Why did you pray so hard for me to live!" She ranted and raved, although at the same time she was terrified that she'd end up all alone like her roommate, who never had visitors. But Laura wouldn't abide it. She told Jessica to stop crying, that she wouldn't come to see her if she was going to be full of self-pity.

One night, about two weeks into treatment, they ended up sharing a good cry together and hugging each other for twenty minutes. Laura stroked her daughter's hair, and Jessica fell asleep in her arms. The crying, at least for that night, stopped, as Jessica drifted off into the best night's sleep she'd had in weeks. Seeing how helpful it was to Jessica to be allowed to give voice to her fears, the team came to better understand the types of interventions that would help her more quickly gain control of her other emotions. Thereafter, Jessica was specifically asked by the staff to discuss her feelings.

As Jessica's behavioral plan took shape, it came to also involve reengineering her environment to reduce distractions and noisy confusion. Although she was not able to comprehend a point system, the staff implemented a procedure known as "time out on the spot." When Jessica erupted with irrational emotions, she would be guided to her chair and everyone except her supervising therapist would leave the room. All background noise would cease (to help her focus), and no further conversations would be held with her until she regained control of herself. Soon Jessica began to recognize that this on-the-spot isolation was associated with her outbursts; she learned to stop herself before the need for the protocol was required. Since she was such a social person, having the silent observation of her therapist also drove the point home that such behavior would not help her meet her goal of getting nurturing interactions.

However, it must be emphasized that in the early days after this protocol was implemented, her behavior actually got worse. I can't stress this point enough, because the result at first seemed so contradictory to achieving the goal it was designed to accomplish. The explanation that I gave to Laura, and the one that I still usually give to families, likens the situation to the trauma of ending the 2 A.M. feeding of a baby. Once the baby's mother—who is on the brink of exhaustion—and the pediatrician have determined that the 2 A.M. feeding is no longer necessary for the health of the infant, it is time for it to stop. Yet, no one can tell a baby that the rules have suddenly changed, so she still cries as usual at 2 A.M. Of course, everyone in the house is awakened, and it becomes painful to hear the continuing cries from the nursery. But, if on that first night, the family can wait it out, eventually the infant goes back to sleep (even if the other members of the household do not). Very likely, after a few nights, the baby will no longer wake up and cry at 2 A.M. But if you get up and give in that first night, just when the pitch of the screaming firmly grabs your guilt-ridden heart, the next night the screaming will start at the new blood-curdling level and it will be even harder to resist continuing the feeding. So, in the end, although those first few nights are very difficult, and initially the infant's screaming gets worse, if you don't respond to it the crying will stop and you will eventually have peaceful nights.

This was exactly the type of behavior that Jessica demonstrated when her plan was started and her cognitive deficits prevented her from understanding the reason for the change. But the staff stuck with the plan every time an outburst occurred, and the result was a decrease in the frequency of Jessica's fits.

As in Jessica's case, successful behavioral therapy can be accomplished with severely impaired patients way before they have achieved any significant cognitive recovery. This is because behavior therapy uses learning pathways that do not require "declarative learning" (see Chapter 12).

Although there are a great number of behavioral interventions that we have not reviewed in this chapter, your introduction to the rehabilitation process is nearly complete. But therapy doesn't stop when your loved one is discharged from formal rehabilitation. There is another whole part of the rehabilitation process, the one that must be continued and generalized into real life, once the goal of returning home has been reached. This is the real test of any rehabilitation program—its ability to prepare a person and his family for the real world, which is filled with even more challenges and frustrations than the patient can imagine at a joyful discharge conference.

On this "nonprosthetic" environment, behavioral outbursts are just not tolerated, end of story; they can bring the police to the door. (And showing a medic alert bracelet imprinted with "I'm brain-injured" is not a get-out-of-jail-free card.) Incomplete assignments cannot simply be reassigned—a failing grade is recorded in an academic transcript. And no one is going to walk on eggshells just so a brain-injured individual won't have to experience stress.

Yet, with loving family and a good treatment team, a brain-injured person can manage well. Hope must never be lost.

PART 4

The Journey Back

chapter 14

REENTERING THE REAL WORLD

> *I like myself better now!*
> —Leigh Ann Jones, TBI survivor

In 2006, CBS-TV news interviewed forty-year-old Sarah Scantin. At the age of eighteen, she had been hit by a drunken driver and then was run over by a second car. Diagnosed with a severe TBI, she wasn't expected to live. But she did. And after several weeks in a coma, she woke up. For the next fourteen years, she stayed in a minimally conscious state with low awareness of her surroundings. After years of being cared for in a long-term specialty medical hospital, she suddenly began to speak. That day she called her brother on the telephone and said hello.

I applaud such stories and, in my twenty-five-plus years in the world of brain-injury rehabilitation, I have seen them firsthand. *But they are the exceptions to the rule.* And that can be a bitter pill for the majority of families to take. Most of my patients don't have sudden breakthroughs but instead make slow but steady progress over months or even years. Rarely is the trajectory of recovery an upwardly progressing straight line. More often, recovery resembles the upward side of a cross-cut saw: a few steps forward, some backsliding, and then more slow progress.

Let's take a more in-depth look at how a few of the people who were in-troduced in earlier chapters have fared over time on their journey from in-jury to reentry into their new lives.

Take Bruce Robertson, for example, the severely brain-damaged young man who was in a horrific car accident in the Nevada desert. When the ambulance got him to the closest hospital forty-five minutes away, he was in a deep coma. He had flat-lined, but was resuscitated by the time he got to the trauma center, where he lay in a coma for over two weeks. His doc-tors told his family not to expect him to get better—that if he came out of the coma at all, he would have severe deficits.

And he did—at first. When he came out of his coma, he screamed and flailed his arms. His mother, Mary Ann, if you remember, laid herself on top of him for forty-eight hours to stop him from hurting himself. Bruce's par-ents were told they should look for a nursing home where he could live out the remainder of his life. But his mother wouldn't have any of it; she wanted him home. "When they told me he wouldn't get out of the coma, I told them he would—and he did. When they told me he wouldn't get any better than a vegetative state, I told them he would—and he did."

He did better than that. For his one year in a neurospecialty facility, he and his rehab team worked hard to teach him compensatory strategies. In this setting, all of the handicapping conditions—that is, the disabilities af-fecting both his physical and his cognitive/behavioral problems—were managed well enough so that he could go home. His physical deficits were actually much easier to manage than those associated with impaired self-awareness and the uncontrollable anger that appeared whenever he needed redirection because of his poor safety judgment. His mom hired a nurse technician that Bruce called "Hertz-Rent-a-Buddy." He took Bruce on errands and reminded him of things he might have forgotten.

After about three years, Bruce was able to volunteer at the facility where he'd been a patient. He helped patients with skills training, outings, and vocational training. He even lectured on brain-injury prevention at local high schools and received a degree as a certified medical assistant.

As of this writing, thirteen years later, Bruce has married and holds a steady job, as you may recall, as an apartment-complex manager. His anger is managed with both behavioral strategies and medication.

As fate would have it, Bruce's mother was in a car accident six years after Bruce's accident. At the hospital, Mary Ann was diagnosed with broken bones, along with damage to her pelvis and bladder. The injuries were so severe that she had to stay in a long-term acute-care hospital for three months to recuperate. After she was discharged, her husband showed her photographs he'd taken of her in the hospital. One look at the pictures told her that she had had a brain injury, too. "I could see it in my face, in my eyes. My son had had the same look, like something was slightly off or just not there."

Mary Ann came to see me. A detailed history of her acute injury, coupled with a battery of exploratory tests, confirmed her self-diagnosis. She had experienced a moderately severe diffuse hypoxemic or anoxic brain injury. Today, her short-term memory remains impaired, but she gets by with the help of a personal journal and detailed checklists.

After Leah Roberts's stroke in 2004, her family was told she would have severe deficits. At first, the predictions appeared correct. She had partial paralysis on her right side, she couldn't walk, and she couldn't speak. She knew, in her mind, what she wanted to say, but she couldn't get it out. She'd look at people, hear them speak, and understand what they said— but she couldn't respond. She felt trapped in her own head.

Following her initial hospitalization and three months of outpatient rehabilitation, she not only could speak reasonably clearly but also got her old job back as a secretary in the human resources department of a Texas company. No, she is not the "old Leah," but she is a *new* Leah. With the help of her husband and her sister, through hard work and determination, she has built on her recovery with compensatory strategies that have not left her handicapped. Despite her residual deficits, she can now put words to her thoughts and communicate her needs, and she has relearned how to problem-solve at work to accomplish her duties.

She has also learned to overcome the right-sided paralysis to the point where it is difficult to notice her limp. Her walking has been improved by a specially fitted brace worn on the lower leg and foot to support the ankle, hold the foot and ankle in the correct position, and correct foot-drop (known as an ankle-foot orthosis, or *AFO*).

Leah has learned to compensate for her other deficits as well. She avoids noisy malls and large crowds, as the overstimulation easily exhausts her. She keeps a personal journal that contains lists of things to be done each day. Because her immediate short-term memory isn't great, she tends to watch DVDs of movies she's already seen, and reread books that are important to her, to help improve her recall when conversing with friends. .

Leah's employer has also been willing to participate in her recovery by providing reasonable accommodation to ensure her success at work. Leah's coworkers know that they need to e-mail her if they have specific requests. She prints and pastes the requests into her personal journal in a special section to remember what should be incorporated into her "to-do" list. Her journal also contains procedures that she uses on the job. She stays as organized as possible to prevent clutter from distracting her. Because noise and multiple conversations can distract Leah, she closes her door at work when she has to focus on a task. She talks to people one-on-one, never in a group.

To talk to her, you'd hardly know that she'd ever had a severe stroke. "I could never have done this without my sister, Susan," Leah says. "She was with me 24/7. She even helped me take a bath when I wasn't able to do it myself."

Husbands. Wives. Mothers and fathers. Sisters and brothers. All have played integral roles in each of these real-life stories, and it all comes down to one thing: Families can and do have a profound effect on a brain-injured individual's rehabilitation and recovery. That effect can be either very positive, as we have seen in Leah's and Bruce's case, or regrettably negative, as we'll discuss later on in this chapter.

FAMILY FIRST

It's a well-known fact: People with brain injuries do better if they have a supportive family. In one study, it was shown that family involvement leads to significantly lower rates of depression in people with brain injuries, regardless of their severity. Patients with supportive families have been shown to become more effective at problem-solving and can better cope with community reentry after returning home.

In short, there is nothing more powerful than family ties, which can work to a brain-injured person's advantage—or disadvantage. As a whole, families strive to maintain homeostasis—a balance between its members that keeps things safe and secure. There is an instinctual family hierarchy in which everyone—from the cranky breadwinner and the nurturing care-taker to the spoiled brat or the family jokester—has a role to play in maintaining a family's social structure, either enhancing or subtracting from its necessary cohesiveness.

This hierarchy is dynamic; it changes as families age, as siblings are born and grow up. But generally, despite temporary setbacks, such as a problem teenager, when there is a crisis families tend to work to restore whatever kind of balance they have achieved over the years they have been together. This is vital for the survival of any family unit and occurs at a very basic, primitive level that is not readily apparent to those involved. A shake-up in a family's homeostasis threatens its continuation, its very survival. This need for balance explains why so many families deny, for example, a teen's obvious drug habit even when it is brought to their attention by a school or law-enforcement agency. It also helps to explain why a family can become so fragile when a caretaker mother decides to get a job and leave the home every day after years of daily devotion to being a successful homemaker.

But when a family member becomes brain-injured, this homeostasis is irrevocably disrupted—with implications that may drive many families apart. Think of it. There is no finality, no death, no moving on. Instead, there are events, an ebb and flow of potential struggle. Prognoses usually change throughout the rehabilitation process; what starts out as a life-threatening emergency becomes an arduous waiting game that feels never-ending. Physical, cognitive, and behavioral rehabilitation continues into the foreseeable future, and a parent may begin to feel that they are little more than a taxi service.

As the rules of the game continue to change with each stage of recovery—as the brain-injured family member comes home from a rehab center, begins community reintegration, or starts vocational training—the family's fragile sense of stability may be threatened again and again. Families may deny that their loved one is different and may resist coming to an emotional understanding of why he can't return to the fast-paced job he once had or why he can't play softball with the kids on the weekends or drive himself to and from the grocery store.

DIFFERENT PEOPLE, DIFFERENT SCENARIOS

So what does reentering the world really mean for a brain-injured individual? Well, the experiences of reentry are as varied as the types of injuries themselves. For the most severely injured, it may mean being able to live in an environment that provides total care while affording privacy, personal dignity, and as much quality of life as possible. It may also mean that families have to either adapt to having their loved one living away from home or turn their own homes into prosthetic environments. This may require, for example, converting a dining room into what resembles an intensive care unit. Some families may feel that this is the only acceptable way for them to feel certain that the long-term needs of their family member are met. Others may feel that such an arrangement would destroy the social fabric of the family, alienating siblings, making everything revolve around the injured family member, and leaving little time for life's other demands.

At the other end of the spectrum, for those 70 to 80 percent of TBI patients with mild brain injuries, life may change little over the long run. However, some form of continuing medical and family management is still necessary during the reentry of these individuals to home, work, or school. In these circumstances, the difficulties are far more subtle but, if left unaddressed, can produce secondary psychosocial problems that only worsen with time. The individual and his family must recognize that short-term accommodation is often necessary in nearly every domain until the cognitive, emotional, and behavioral consequences of MTBI resolve.

For most families, this means ignoring certain behaviors that may be irritating but are not completely disruptive and do not present immediate safety risks. As explained in Chapter 14, by ignoring such behavior, those who are charged with providing care to a brain-injured person avoid reinforcing the behavior and thereby perpetuating it. Caregivers in the family must carefully pick their battles and choose to engage only on issues involving safety. By taking this path, they minimize the risk that everything will become a struggle of wills, which invariably will produce explosions, which in turn are rarely containable until they have run their course.

A few very important limits—such as, "You will not drive the car under any circumstances"; "You will not consume alcohol or drugs while you are living at home with the family"; or "Although you may yell, you will never hit anyone"—should be explicitly stated, written down where they are in view for everyone to see, and strictly enforced, without excuse or question. The question of how to deal with violations of these agreements then becomes of paramount importance. The best advice that I have come up with over the past twenty-five years has been to speak with local authorities regarding their willingness to help your family before an incident arises. On occasion, a letter from a physician may strengthen your hand in engaging them to intervene. The risk of a physical encounter escalating out of control to the point where someone could get hurt is so high in these circumstances that it is wise to have law-enforcement backup to ensure safety. It has been my experience that the brain-injured person may test this arrangement once, but if it works as planned, it is rarely, if ever, needed in the future.

Patients in the middle group—those with moderately severe brain injuries—often present the greatest challenges upon returning home. In these circumstances, both physical and behavioral accommodations are required for successful reentry. Planning for the return home must begin while the individual is still being cared for at a rehabilitation facility. The first step is to have a specially trained member of the interdisciplinary treatment team come to the home to do a formal "home assessment." This involves evaluating the home to determine whether renovations will be needed to accommodate the width of wheelchairs, for example, or to facilitate an individual's ability to safely transfer from a wheelchair to the commode or shower (through the use of bars to hold onto, shower chairs, and the like). If there are stairs leading into the home, a ramp may need to be added.

The rehab team can usually recommend local vendors who are able to perform the modifications to the home correctly and at a reasonable cost, as such accommodations are very unlikely to be paid for by external funding sources. However, I have seen community groups or members of a religious community volunteer their services to help when funding is scarce.

The home evaluation also involves assessing the items in the home that may be dangerous to someone who has safety-judgment difficulties. Many of these dangers are in the kitchen, involving stoves, toaster ovens, and the like. The therapist will usually recommend the storage of special or valuable objects that might get broken, as brain-injured people often have balance problems that make them unable to safely handle such objects.

The Role of the Treatment Team

The next phase of preparing for reentry involves having the family regularly attend interdisciplinary treatment planning conferences. The family needs to begin to understand the various areas of disability and the current focus of treatment. What is being done in each area (physical and neurological, cognitive, social, and so on) to accomplish realistic goals? As the patient moves back to the home, the family must be brought on board to support those objectives and given the information they need to understand what they can do to help. It is now time for the family to work with the case manager, the program director, and the social worker to set up specific times when they can attend treatment sessions to learn how the therapists approach the injured family member's remaining deficits.

It is vital for the family to learn these strategies and to emulate them as closely as possible when helping the patient with activities such as showering, dressing, and transferring from a wheelchair to a car seat, commode, or dinner table. Consistency helps the patient proceduralize these activities so that they can become a part of his motor memory, which will allow him to perform them without having to think about the steps of the process. Having to actively think about everything one must do is exhausting for an injured patient at this stage of recovery and cannot be sustained for any realistic period of time. When the same steps are repeated over and over, the activity becomes routinized into a reliable behavioral change.

The physical and occupational therapists should develop a home program for family members to help the patient with on a daily basis, even if outpatient physical therapy (PT) and occupational therapy (OT) are planned. These home programs help to reinforce the body mechanics necessary to correctly perform various activities of daily living and reduce the chance of the patient developing maladaptive patterns of movement that produce their own set of problems. Many patients want to do things their own way—or want to avoid their home exercises—to reduce discomfort, but this can hinder the development of skill sets that lay the foundation for later progress. Conditioning exercises are generally recommended to build endurance, for example, so that performing daily routines will become less fatiguing with time. Many patients complain that they are "just too tired" to do these exercises, but if the family caregivers permit these activities to be set aside, the fatigue will only get worse, and the patient will be able to do less and less as time goes on. The only way to overcome fatigue is to work at becoming stronger so that each activity takes less total energy to perform.

Family caregivers also benefit greatly from working with staff at this stage to observe how they handle episodes of maladaptive behavior. This is one of the most difficult areas for families to master, given the differences between the relationships a patient has with rehab staff members and the relationships he has with his family members. Old behavioral patterns often govern family interactions, and these long-established habits are difficult to break. Of course, there are those uncanny ways that family members have of provoking one another that they may not even be conscious of after the years or decades over which they have developed. The goal for family members is to try to depersonalize many of the kinds of interactions that may have been such an active part of their preinjury lives.

It is vital for the family to work with the medical staff to understand any medications that will need to be administered at home. Family members need to know when generic substitutions are acceptable and what side effects to watch for. They will be charged with making sure that the patient takes her medications in the right doses and on time. The medication schedule should be clearly posted, and pills should be kept in a pill container that helps everyone keep track of the dosages for each day and times of day. On occasion, a family member may have to actually check to verify that the patient has actually swallowed her medications, as, in some cases, patients are not willing to comply. Be sure to ask the doctor what to do if a dose is missed, because some medications can be taken more often to make up for missed doses, while others cannot.

Family members also need to know how to recognize the difference between a true allergy to a medication and an adverse reaction. A true allergy is always associated with hives that cover the palms of the hands and the soles of the feet and produce itching. On occasion, shortness of breath may accompany the rash, and this constitutes an emergency requiring immediate medical attention. Breathing problems can be fatal, so an allergic reaction of this type warrants a trip to the closest emergency room or a 911 call for help. On the other hand, many of us have adverse reactions to medications—typically, nausea or vomiting. These symptoms are not signs of allergies, and in some circumstances the drug can still be used while the side effects are managed.

Family caregivers should make sure they have all the necessary prescriptions either in hand or phoned in prior to discharge in order to prevent lapses in dosing. Also, it is best to work with the staff to get all outpatient appointments set up prior to discharge, as it can take a while to get in to see some physicians on an outpatient basis. Whenever possible, the caregiver should ask for copies of the neuroimaging studies; often they can be provided on a CD or DVD to be kept at home and used for later comparison when similar studies are ordered on an outpatient basis. Although your physician will also keep them on file, it is still a good idea to have an extra copy for the radiologist to refer to later on.

Finally, families must have the ability to safely transport an injured family member back and forth—whether it is to therapy sessions, doctor's appointments, or just everyday outings that the patient is capable of enjoying. If a wheelchair is involved and the patient cannot safely transfer from the chair to a car seat independently, or even with the help of others, the family may need to purchase a specialized van. The van should be equipped

TEN PREDICTORS

The following factors may lead to better recovery outcomes for a brain-injured person (although it is not a definitive list—patients with all of these factors in their favor may not do as well as expected, and patients without them may still do quite well over the long term):

1. A less severe injury
2. Preinjury native intelligence, motivation, and resilience
3. Lack of preinjury risk-taking behavior or drug or alcohol abuse
4. A prior history of successful accomplishment at home, work, or school
5. An employer or school district that is willing to accommodate special needs
6. Local authorities who recognize the possible need for help in maintaining the safety of the family and home
7. The ability of the family and patient to adjust to new realities, sometimes termed **cognitive flexibility** and **behavioral malleability**
8. Financial aid and monetary resources
9. Community and workplace ties
10. Family support

with a specially installed lift to ensure safe transport. Many of the therapies discussed in this book may need to be continued on an outpatient basis to provide for a smooth transition from the controlled, prosthetic environment of a rehab facility to the understandably more loosely organized life at home.

Families should expect a period of adjustment for all concerned once the brain-injured member returns home. Often, just following discharge, there is a brief "honeymoon period" (of perhaps two weeks) where everything seems to be going so well as to make the family wonder if all that preparation for reentry was really necessary. Soon, however, as the novelty wears off, everyone begins to assume that things should be getting back to normal again. Then, when the inevitable problems arise, patience may give way to regular irritation, and some family members come to resent all the time and attention that is needed to care for the brain-injured loved one at home. Children, in particular, have a hard time subordinating their needs to those of an injured sibling and become increasingly needy themselves. Generally, this is when it becomes important to make sure everyone gets a break from time to time. A grandparent or an aunt or uncle can take the siblings out to do something special, for example, or come in to care for the injured family member so that the rest of the nuclear family can have some time alone.

BACK TO WORK, SCHOOL, OR SOCIAL ACTIVITY

Once life has returned to some kind of predictable pattern, it is time to take the next steps toward community entry and social integration. For the most severely impaired individuals, it may be extremely difficult to resume the activities that were once a large part of their lives, either at work or school. In that case, caregivers must look for venues outside the home where the individual may have time to be with other people and form new relationships.

Some of these settings may be sponsored by local brain-injury support groups; others may occur at community centers that provide outreach for individuals with different types of disabilities; still others may take place in conjunction with a local school or religious organization. The trick here is to not just make a one-shot appearance; only by regular attendance can the brain-injured individual develop the beginnings of the kinds of relationships with other participants that may lead to friendship and ultimately close companionship. This process can take months, so the caregiver must not be discouraged if first encounters do not produce the desired results. The development of any relationship takes time, and this is especially true for someone who has sustained a severe brain injury.

For those with mild injuries, all that may be required for reintegration to work or school to begin is to merely let the organization know what has occurred as a result of the injury. Under these circumstances, most employers and all school districts will provide reasonable accommodation to help the transition occur smoothly. Some school districts may have special forms that need to be filled out by a licensed physician, and most require a conference with the family to review the student's current circumstances and the likely impact of the disabilities on her participation in classroom and extracurricular activities.

For those with moderately severe brain injuries, returning to work or school may become a more complicated affair. For adults, this is the time when I am interested in having both formal neuropsychological testing and a structured vocational evaluation performed. If there are any questions about driving, and no medical contraindications, such as an active seizure disorder or ongoing memory problems, a state-certified driving evaluation must be conducted prior to permitting any patient to drive. This is nonnegotiable, as the risks to the injured individual as well as to society are extremely high.

The goal of well-performed neuropsychological testing that clearly correlates its findings with the patient's clinical history is to give everyone concerned an idea of the individual's relative cognitive strengths and weaknesses. The information obtained from neuropsychological testing, particularly that which clearly identifies a patient's residual cognitive strengths, must also be correlated with information from her vocational testing. The vocational testing itself helps to identify the person's skills from preinjury work experiences and suggests jobs that she may find interesting and rewarding. Finally, all this information can be pieced together and matched with the types of jobs that are available near the patient's home, and a plan can be created that attempts to find actual paid employment opportunities for the patient. The goal is to find positions that the patient has the highest possible likelihood of being successful in performing. Nothing is gained by encouraging a brain-injury survivor to return to work in a position where he is likely to fail. Success builds upon success, so the first experience at reemployment postinjury must be carefully chosen.

In some circumstances, I may request that a "job coach" act as a liaison with the patient's employer to help ease the transition back to work. This coach can help identify potential problems before they mushroom into issues that can threaten the patient's potential for continued employment in the chosen job. Sometimes, a job coach will actually work side by side with the survivor until the routines of his job are firmly established. Over time, the brain-injured individual can perform the job successfully with less and less help, and the job coach can gradually extricate herself from the day-to-day activities of the job. The coach remains available to both the survivor and his employer should problems arise.

For students, most school districts have a very structured process to help ease a child's return to school. At first, a teacher may come to the home and help the student get restarted in coursework without the social pressures of being at school. School testing and family meetings are held along the way, and a plan evolves to return the student to the classroom, often with special accommodations. His progress is routinely assessed, and the school plan is adjusted accordingly. Behavioral problems may need specialized treatment to prevent them from precluding full reintegration into the classroom.

The areas addressed in this chapter are only some of the issues that must be taken into consideration when planning for a successful transition from treatment back into the real world. However, what is most important for the family to know is that such a journey can successfully occur when appropriate planning is started early in the course of rehabilitation. Although the individual's life may not be the same as the one he had prior to the injury, life can continue, and fulfillment remains a possibility.

Sigmund Freud defined a good life as having the ability to both love and work. Theories may come and go, but truths such as this one remain constant throughout the ages.

chapter 15

TAKING CARE OF THE CAREGIVER — YOU

Love yourself—accept yourself—forgive
yourself—and be good to yourself, because
without you the rest of us are without a source
of many wonderful things.
—Leo F. Buscaglia

One day, as I was on an elevator heading off to lunch after presiding over a family treatment conference, I had an eye-opening experience. The patient I had just been conferring about was a young man who had experienced a severe TBI and was now six weeks' post injury. He had not yet had a return of continuous memory and was unable to perform any of the activities of ordinary daily life without a great deal of assistance from the staff. Two team members were often required to help transfer him from one place to another. Up until quite recently, he had been unable to self-regulate the amount of food he put in his mouth at one time, placing him at risk of aspiration. But he had made progress, and we felt that we could reduce the amount of supervision with his meals. Crowded in the back of an elevator, I noticed the young man's parents squash themselves in just as the doors were closing. They had no idea I was in the back and began talking about their experience of the meeting we had just concluded.

The patient's mother couldn't understand what the rehab team was so excited about. The father responded, "I agree. They're all charged up about him being able to eat his own lunch with only one person helping, and what I really wanted to know was: When is he going back to work?"

Thus began my education as to how different a family's views may be from those of the staff. We who work in the field of neurorehabilitation can become completely detached from what the patient's family is experiencing during the recovery. Instead of taking the time to put the patient's recovery in perspective for the family, we had assumed they would understand how long rehabilitation would take. We saw the small, incremental changes we knew would eventually add up to a "reasonable outcome" from severe brain injury. We were focused on the "trees," but the family needed to hear more about the "forest" they were living in with their family member. I began to understand that one of my main responsibilities to every family is to help them realize that although we cannot yet cure brain injury, we do have a general idea of the path the recovering person must travel before coming out of that forest of confusion; it goes hand in hand that along with the rest of the staff I must attempt to make the bumpy, obstacle-ridden trail ahead easier to navigate.

If there's one thing I've learned over the years—and I hope it's become clear in this book—it's that every brain-injury case is different, but patterns do emerge with time, and wisdom comes from experience. Each physical injury is unique. Each person sustaining an injury to the brain is biologically and psychologically unique as well, and the life circumstances that each one brings to the injury from past experiences are a part of a unique life story. The statement "the whole is greater than the sum of its parts" comes to mind. When all these variables are added together, the result forms yet another new and unique pattern. But although it is unique, it is not inscrutable. Let's call this new pattern "the Big Picture."

It is this "Big Picture," as well as the individual components of the picture, that a physician must consider when treating brain injury. The individual components of the picture interact with each other as well as with "the Big Picture" itself. This interaction can have significant effects on treatment planning and outcome. The individual components that a physician must keep up with and be mindful of include what is going on in each domain—the physical, the psychological, and the psychosocial—to the best of his ability, to provide appropriate treatment recommendations in each that will impact "the Big Picture" as time goes on—preventing what can be prevented and treating what will ultimately remain.

One of the most important components of "the Big Picture" is you—a member of the family of the brain-injured person. It is from this perspective that I approach the topic of this chapter, which is to offer suggestions to caregivers as to how they can take care of themselves while still caring for their loved one. To all the caretakers who are reading this book, keeping "the Big Picture" in mind, please understand that there is no magic pill, book, relaxation exercise, therapeutic intervention, or support group that is guaranteed to effectively address the complex, individual needs that you, also a unique individual, may have, any more than there is only one effective treatment for brain injury itself. The physician must carefully consider "the Big Picture" when addressing the needs of the caregiver, just as she does when addressing the needs of the patient.

Having said this, I realize that these initial observations may be of little comfort to you as a caregiver who is seeking guidance as to how you may better cope with your circumstances. But in an effort to address your needs, while being mindful of "the Big Picture," I asked myself this question: After over a quarter of a century of working with brain-injured patients and their families, what are the top five pieces of general advice that I can offer to family members regarding their own well-being as they make their own individual journey through the ordeal of coping with brain injury? After much deliberation, I decided on the following suggestions, and I sincerely hope they are of some benefit to you.

1. TAKE ONE STEP AT A TIME

Individual rates and courses of recovery differ from one individual to the next owing to multiple, and often unpredictable, variables. Keep "the Big Picture" in mind. A change in one domain of a patient's condition can alter it, sometimes for the better and sometimes for the worse. If it's for the worse, don't get discouraged. The change may be temporary, or a change in another domain may yet again change the picture—this time for the better. Take one step at a time. Don't write a life script based on one snapshot in time.

It is difficult to not overreact to moment-to-moment and day-to-day crises that your family member may experience. Experienced physicians and rehabilitation teams don't put too much stock in any one day or any one event, but rather step back and look at what trends are developing. Changing a treatment plan based on every momentary change or "fluke" that a patient may experience wreaks havoc on all concerned. Often, the "tincture of time" is the best solution. Erratic therapeutic changes can be very harmful and produce their own complications that can cloud "the Big Picture." Medications take time to work. The introduction of true behavioral therapy may lead to transient increases in maladaptive behavior, and inconsistent, off-the-cuff explanations of what is going on will only make you more confused. This is not to say that changes in treatment plans will not occur—of course they will, as time progresses—but making those changes is like playing a three-dimensional chess game: Each modification must be carefully thought out as recovery evolves.

2. DON'T EXPECT ANY GUARANTEES—GOOD OR BAD

As you and your family make the journey toward recovery, be realistic. Keep the flame of hope alive in your heart that the very best possible outcome may occur for your family member, but don't let that hope overshadow your grasp of reality. No one can guarantee you an ideal outcome.

On the other hand, just because things start looking bad, that doesn't mean that your family member is guaranteed a bad outcome. Beware of people who speak in such absolutes. Such attitudes may indicate nothing more than a person's limitations in understanding the complexities of brain-injury treatment.

Families dealing with brain injury are bombarded with so many different opinions about what they should do. Some of these views will be extreme, and both ends of the spectrum can be dangerous. Keep in mind that many of the people who give you advice don't know what they don't know. A great many of them are well-meaning people, but they sometimes forcefully push their opinions without realizing that they have missed an entire area of consideration and based their conclusions on erroneous assumptions. This is where wisdom must be exercised. At times, the best answer you can give such people is "Thank you for your ideas; I'll consider them carefully and talk to our doctor about it."

3. REMEMBER THAT YOU AND YOUR LOVED ONE ARE UNIQUE

No two injuries are identical. No two people are identical. Even identical twins are not exactly the same, as they have different experiences throughout their lives. No two families are identical. No two treatment programs are the same. You and your injured family member have a relationship that is like no other.

With all of these unique factors to consider in every case, no one can tell you exactly how things will turn out for your loved one. An experienced rehabilitation team must be prepared to discuss the probabilities of the various outcomes in your situation. Although this uncertainty may at first make you feel uncomfortable, it is the rule rather than the exception, that each stage of recovery has a variety of possible outcomes. Treatment approaches that work for one patient may be useless or even detrimental when applied to another. Your big picture is unique and must be viewed as such in treatment planning.

Although many elements of brain-injury treatment and rehabilitation are standardized according to evidence-based medicine, excellent treatment involves the proper blending of these different elements to fit the circumstances of each individual. Be wary of "cookie-cutter" programs with teams that do not have routine, daily experience in neurorehabilitation. Neurorehabilitation is *not* the same as general physical medicine and rehabilitation. Programs that work with fractured hips, spinal cord injuries, sports medicine, and the like rarely see enough neurorehabilitation patients to permit them to focus specifically on the unique factors of brain-injury rehabilitation. Thus, often these programs focus on what is seen as a consequence of the injury, not what has truly happened to the brain that produces both what is seen and unseen.

Finally, any program that claims it can do everything for everyone rarely, if ever, does anything very well.

4. AVOID ISOLATION AND TAKE TIME FOR YOURSELF

At the beginning of a traumatic event, people are usually coming out of the woodwork to offer their help and assistance. It's just human nature, as most of us acutely feel the pain that our friends and extended family members are going through at the start of any crisis. However, unlike many other diseases and illnesses, brain injury is not one that gets a quick fix—a few days in the hospital and then a person is as good as new. Recovering from severe brain injury is a grueling experience that will wear anyone down, no matter how tough you may think you are.

For most families, it is very hard to leave the ICU when an injured family member is still in immediate danger—yet, at this point in time, when his "computer" (brain) is completely "unplugged," he will have no memory of the events that whirled around him, ever. Most hospitals have rules that restrict family visits to the ICU to just fifteen minutes every one to two hours. To anxious family members, those brief but precious visits are priceless, and most people feel compelled to wait for each and every one of them. This is understandable, of course, but continuing the so-called "coma vigil" for weeks will inevitably cause you to "hit the wall" and burn yourself out.

My recommendation is that once you have a general level of comfort with the staff and the environment, you let those willing friends and other family members come and spell you—so that you can get some well-deserved rest. Make sure you also get enough time to exercise your own body—even if you didn't exercise regularly before—because sitting around through this vigil will decondition you, making it physically harder to get through each day.

I can also assure you that despite their best intentions, most of those initial well-wishers will stop coming by as time goes on and their own

worlds begin to consume them once again. Setting up a visitation schedule can both prevent you from being overwhelmed by the onslaught of
well-wishers and spread out their help so that you will have it when you
need it beyond day one or day two. They will be happy to know they are
doing something to truly help, and you will appreciate the one-on-one
time that they will offer when you may need it most. It may be hard to
imagine, but well-wishers are just as uncomfortable as you are because
they are not sure what to do. Offering structured visitation to all concerned
helps them cope with their own anxieties while reducing your own.

Still, as time goes by and people return to their normal lives, you may
come to feel increasingly isolated and alone. Even spouses rarely have the
same fortitude for visitation, and spending every moment of every day together may push relationships to the breaking point. Now is the time when
you must reach out to other support systems—your community, place of
worship, or other extended family members. If you wait for them to come
to you, you may be disappointed, as no one can read your mind and know
when your needs may be most acute. There are many people who will be
happy to assist you in various ways and provide companionship—once
they know that you need it.

It is also important for your own mental health not to give up all those
activities that have sustained you throughout the years. Going out to dinner, having a "girls' night out," participating in the bowling league, or
making time for community worship can all play their parts, giving you
resting places as you run this marathon.

In addition, most communities offer support groups for families with
brain-injured relatives. You can find such groups by asking your doctor or
by looking in the Yellow Pages or on the Internet. Trying one does not com-
mit you to a lifetime of attendance or to participation in every activity offered. You can see how this experience feels to you and let those feelings
guide your participation. Some of us are group people and some of us just
aren't, so there is no right answer about whether you should sign up with
these organizations.

Individual or family counseling with a trained therapist who has experience with brain injuries may also help you and your family cope with the

enormous changes that are occurring in your lives. Even if other family members are reluctant to go, as a primary caregiver you would be well advised to seek out counseling to help you succeed with the challenges you are facing. Encourage the others to join you, but go on your own if necessary. The stress that you may experience over the next weeks, months, and years can lead to depression and other treatable conditions. Interview a few therapists until you feel comfortable that you are sitting with someone with whom you can form a solid therapeutic relationship. Although any competent and compassionate therapist may help you, I tend to have a gender bias in this area. Over the years, I have found that it may be better to have someone of your own gender help you during such troubling times, as therapy is as much an art as a science.

My concluding thoughts on this topic may be viewed as somewhat controversial, as they pertain to faith. Modern evidence-based medicine does not have all the answers. There is still much that is unknown and even mystifying to us as physicians. Regardless of an individual's spiritual orientation, many people find comfort in the power of prayer. An individual's faith should not be dismissed as non-evidence-based. Rather, it should be respected and acknowledged when viewing that individual's big picture as it pertains to treatment planning and outcome.

5. LIVE IN THE MOMENT

Some things that sound simple, or that have become a cliché, can be much more profound than they at first appear. "Live in the moment" is one of these. On one hand, it is just another aphorism that we hear every day or see again and again in self-help books. In addition, it reflects a concept that is very foreign to most of us. We are either at an age when most of our lives revolve around the past, or we tend to live in anticipation of the future. It is one of those statements that are so easily made, yet so truly hard to actualize in our own lives. I have always been a future-oriented person: Nothing has ever been "good enough," and jumping one hurdle just forces me to set the next one even higher.

Yet, living with my wife through our own experience of her malignant lymphoma and its treatment has forced me to experiment with living more in the moment. No matter how much time I devoted to imagining what would or could come next in my wife's treatment, it was all just a guessing game and an enormous waste of time and worry. I still had to deal with whatever really happened. I have come to learn to suspend my belief that I'm clairvoyant, accept that *I don't know what's going to happen,* and actually wait to hear what the real data are. When I succeed in doing these things, I am better able to live in the moment and not borrow trouble from tomorrow that may not even exist. Accept these thoughts as simple ramblings from one who has been there—they are not a recommendation of a lifestyle, but the ruminations of someone who has finally recognized that he just can't control everything. And neither can you.

Finally, one last thought that may help you deal with the guilt you may experience when you recognize that you just can't do everything for everyone. The reality is that if you burn yourself out and fall ill, your loved one will lose just as much or more than you do. It is in everyone's best interest for you to take care of yourself so that you can successfully complete the marathon that faces you and your family.

Epilogue

THE FUTURE IS NOW

It's been over two centuries since the American Revolution. From the initial shots fired at Bunker Hill in 1775 to this day, approximately 1 million Americans have died in battle. It's been fewer than one hundred years since Henry Ford put the finishing touches on the first mass-produced automobile, but *more than 2.5 million Americans* have died in a car on the road. Today, thanks to modern life-saving techniques, victims are able to survive war wounds, car accidents, and various kinds of other accidents more often than ever before. But, unfortunately, surviving doesn't mean coming back as good as new. Today, there is practically an epidemic of traumatic brain injury—a staggering 6.3 million Americans disabled by TBI.

We don't read about TBI in the daily papers the way we read about heart disease or cancer. It is, in fact, a silent epidemic. Yes, we've made extraordinary inroads in the field of brain science since the "decade of the brain" in the 1990s, but it is the healthy brain that most fascinates us—the areas of the brain that influence memory, that enable a young child to learn so quickly in the first few years of life, or that help us to solve problems or survive tragedy. We've learned how to make our brains smarter, keeping old age at bay; we've learned to strengthen our memory, fine-tune our reactions, and improve our perceptions. And we have learned more about the role of the brain's neurochemistry in addictions, obesity, depression, bipolar disorder, and the like.

But we still aren't sure how to live with TBI.

With all these inroads, all this progress, we still need to rely primarily on symptoms to determine whether someone has had a concussion or a mild head injury. Despite all the advances made in rehabilitation, in understanding the way the brain develops and grows, we still have difficulty accepting behavior as a function of the brain, nothing more and nothing less.

When we break a leg, it's going to affect the way we walk. If we hurt our brain, it's going to affect our behavior. So simple, yet still so difficult for many to grasp. We still mistrust behavior and believe it is completely psychological in nature. We still believe that our severely injured loved ones can be exactly who they were before if they just try hard enough, if we just give them more care, if we just give them one-on-one therapy for twenty weeks.

In the years since I began my practice, we have made progress; there's no doubt about it. But we still have a journey ahead of us, a journey in which we must learn to accept our limitations, the new self born from the remnants of the accident, the stroke, the fall.

The people who come to see me, the patients and their caregivers, work very hard to learn this new way of life. I have always found extraordinary inspiration in them, these unspoken heroes who continue to give when it seems impossible, who keep going when all signs say "stop," who hang on in a world where progress is measured in infinitesimal steps. All of the people you have met in this book have become contributing members of society; they have made peace with their changes and they live fulfilling lives as mothers, fathers, workers, students, and volunteers.

Emily Carter holds down a steady job and is independent enough to drive her own car, and she is a great single mom.

Jessica Collins continues to exercise six days a week and keeps herself fit.

John Lewis is a great grandfather and husband, and he's found that he has a talent for landscaping.

Leah Roberts is back at her old job in human resources and she's been welcomed with open arms.

Chris Barron is happier than he ever was; he's a top executive at his company and he travels regularly to the Middle East.

Mary Ann Robertson gets to see her son, Bruce, more than before; he lives with his wife and children and he still works successfully managing his apartment complex, getting plenty of time to work outdoors.

Y. J. Ming has gotten off the treadmill and has a quiet life that includes more golf. He and his wife now have two beautiful kids, and they've never known their dad any other way.

John Stambino has started composing music again.

Troy Atkins is a freshman in college and doing well.

Louise McDougal and her family are learning new ways to communicate. She laughs a lot more than she did when she first came to our hospital.

And Sam O'Connell? He's hugging his baby son as we speak.

Are they different? Sure. And, like all of us, they have their good days and their bad. But they are functioning, living their lives, becoming parents, working and earning money. They are loved.

I wrote this book for these people and for all of my patients, to help them better help themselves. By allowing me to tell their stories, they have made an impact. I hope you, too, will become inspired, and that you will learn something from this book to help in your battle with TBI.

Whenever any of us have had no prior experience in a specialty area, its complexities seem endless. This is especially true in brain injury, as no one ever volunteers; everyone is drafted. If you have read this far, by now you know that the body of knowledge that exists about TBI is as finite as any other. We all need professional help and coaches to help us find our way in some areas of our lives. I could never replace the transmission in my own car; I go to my mechanic for that. Likewise, if your loved one has suffered a brain injury, you will need help navigating the confusing symptoms, complex therapies, and many different sorts of rehabilitation services ahead of you. Consider this book to be your portable coach as you work to help your loved one take her first tentative steps back into life.

I always say, "Prepare for the worst, but expect the best." Because in every scenario, there is some light, however slim; there is some hope. We can fight the aftermath of TBI together because hope never dies.

Neither does progress.

And neither does love.

Appendix: How the Brain Works

> *If the human brain were so simple that we could understand it, we would be so simple that we couldn't.*
>
> —Emerson M. Pugh

If you've turned to this section, you're looking for a more detailed understanding of how the brain works. To that end, we will begin by reviewing the entire human nervous system, over which the brain reigns supreme, just as if we were going from New York City to Los Angeles.

First, we'll see how the nerves that run throughout our entire bodies, usually in parallel with our blood vessels, form what is known as the *peripheral nervous system (PNS)*. The PNS is responsible for transmitting information from our bodies to the *central nervous system (CNS)*, which consists of the spinal cord and the brain, and vice versa. It keeps the CNS informed of external bodily information, on the one hand, and gets information back to the body from the CNS on how to effectively respond to these environmental changes, on the other.

Next, we will review how the human *skull* encases the brain, much like a helmet covers our heads, and how the spinal column is not only responsible for producing reflexive reactions that keep us out of harm's way but also for collecting the massive amount of sensory information from our

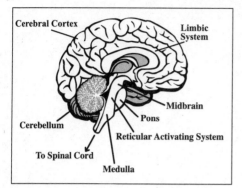

Figure A-1   Side view of brain, including brainstem, limbic system, cerebellum, and cerebral cortex

bodies. The spinal cord must then tightly compact this information, as well as the brain's instructions back to the body, so that these pathways can fit through a rather small, roughly circular opening at the base of the skull called the *foramen magnum.* This vital connection transitions and links the functions of the spinal cord to the human brain. It is useful to recall that the most basic brain functions, from an evolutionary perspective, are its most primitive. This most primitive part of the human brain is known as the *brain stem.* Historically, the human brain has been roughly divided into three major components: the brain stem, which includes the pons and midbrain; the limbic system; and the cerebral cortex.

The brain stem comprises four major structures: the *medulla oblongata,* the *reticular activating system,* the *pons,* and the *midbrain.* These areas of the brain are responsible for the most basic functions necessary for human survival, such as regulation of heart and breathing rates, maintenance of normal blood pressure, and control over general arousal as well as sleep-wake cycles. Most of the specialized *cranial nerves* come from the brain stem. The cranial nerves are specialized sensory and motor nerve tracts that send information to and from the brain; for example, the second cranial nerve, named the *optic nerve,* transmits visual information from our eyes to the brain.

Then, we will explore the *limbic system,* generally viewed as consisting of the structures that contain our memories and generate many of our emotional responses. These are the areas of the brain that are also responsible for the production of certain primitive behavioral traits, such as sexuality, aggression, and territoriality as well as parental protectiveness of offspring.

The *cerebral cortex,* sometimes referred to as the *neocortex,* is the layer of the brain often called *gray matter.* The cortex is gray because nerves in this area lack the insulation (*myelin*) that makes most other parts of the brain appear to be white. It is about one to two inches thick and covers the outer portions of the brain. The cerebral cortex consists of folded bulges called *gyri* that create deep furrows, or fissures, called *sulci*. The folding of the brain is functionally designed to increase its surface area without increasing its overall size, thereby permitting the evolution of increasingly sophisticated brain associations that involve literally millions of connections throughout the brain. The cerebral cortex is divided into right and left hemispheres and is the most recently evolved structure of the human brain. It's the part of the brain that forms the basis of what makes us most uniquely human.

Finally, we'll review the structure and function of the cells that make up the brain, the information-transporting *neurons* and their support cells, which are known as *glial cells.*

THE PERIPHERAL NERVOUS SYSTEM

The peripheral nervous system (PNS) consists of all the nerves outside of the spinal cord and brain. Nerves and blood vessels usually travel together throughout our bodies. These nerves carry information to and from the central nervous system (brain and spinal cord) that direct most bodily functions, from moving our arms to controlling our bladders. In order for the brain to acquire information about the environment, it is vital for the PNS to work properly and for the spinal cord to be fully intact. Likewise, the brain must respond to this information to keep the body safe and functioning properly. For example, if the PNS informs the brain that the body is cold, the brain sends multiple messages back to the PNS, causing our blood vessels to constrict and the muscles of the body to begin shivering (producing heat). The brain's most sophisticated feedback is what causes us to go get a coat and gives us the coordination needed to put it on.

THE SKULL AND PROTECTIVE MEMBRANES

The peripheral nervous system and the spinal cord are ultimately responsible for getting information transmitted throughout the body. They join the

BRAIN DRAIN 101

If you are caring for a loved one who has had a brain injury, you might feel a little overwhelmed by some of the new words you'll be hearing from health-care professionals. The list below should help.

- The areas of bruising and bleeding on the surface of the brain are called **contusions.**
- An **anterior,** or **ventral,** injury is one that occurs toward the front of the head.
- A **posterior,** or **dorsal,** injury occurs to the back of the head.
- Higher structures are referred to as **rostral** (toward the head) and lower ones are called **caudal** (toward the feet).
- **Lateral** refers to the side of the brain, and **medial** refers to the center or middle.
- If an injury is confined to one particular area, it is known as a **focal injury.**
- If an injury occurs across the entire brain, it's called **diffuse.**
- When nerve cells are damaged and the connections between one part of the brain and another are either torn or chemically broken, it's called a **diffuse axonal injury.**

brain at the base of the skull. There are basically two structures of the head to consider in brain injuries: the skull and the brain. To understand brain injury, we must have a basic knowledge about how the skull both protects, and also may harm, the brain.

The skull is made of bone that has a protective function for the brain. In ordinary life, the skull prevents injury to the brain from the effects of many minor traumas that involve the head. The brain itself has the consistency of Jell-O. The skull evolved to prevent harm to the brain from blunt trauma, such as a creature might experience by, say, running into a tree. However, for humans, the world has very quickly (at least in evolutionary terms) become much more complex than it was in prehistoric or ancient times, or even than it was a hundred years ago, especially with the invention of motor vehicles, which routinely accelerate our heads and our brains to speeds of sixty-five or seventy miles per hour. The skull was never designed to protect the brain from the abrupt deceleration that occurs with a fall of more than six feet or with the impact from a serious car accident. The rigid bony structures stop moving much more quickly than the gelatinous brain matter inside, which is essentially trapped within the bony skull. This difference in composition permits the brain to bounce back and forth like a Ping-Pong ball until it finally comes to rest. Ironically, the skull actually contributes to the injuries caused by rapid deceleration, because the brain continues to move once the heavier and denser skull has stopped. In essence, what was meant to shield the brain (the skull) can actually cause it harm.

If you could look at the inside of the skull with the top bones removed, you would see the bony structures that can injure the brain in acceleration-deceleration traumatic brain injuries. The largest opening in the skull is called the *foramen magnum* and it is another danger zone. The foramen magnum is where the spinal cord and the brain connect in the area of the brain stem. If a brain injury produces increased pressure on the brain, the brain stem may be pushed through this opening, often leading to death.

Just beneath the skull, the brain is covered with three membranes. The first and toughest is the *dura*. The other two layers of membranes are the *pia*, a thin lining that hugs the brain, and the *arachnoid*, a web-like lining covering the pia. In the event of a brain injury, these membranes can also be damaged; blood can collect between each layer, further complicating the damage. The most life-threatening type of bleeding is known as an *epidural hematoma*, because this often leads to herniation of the brain stem through the foramen magnum.

The brain is encased in a fluid called *cerebrospinal fluid (CSF)*. This clear liquid nourishes and protects the brain like an air bag in a car. It fills open spaces in the brain called *ventricles* and is replenished with new fluid six times a day. When the brain is damaged, blood may clot and block the outflow of cerebrospinal fluid into the spinal canal. If this occurs, the CSF may build up and add damaging pressure to the injury. Often, this can only be corrected by placing a shunt into the brain (often referred to as an *intraventricular peritoneal shunt*) that drains the fluid into the abdomen. The CSF also bathes the inner membranous covering of the brain.

THE BRAIN STEM AND ITS CONNECTIONS

The brain stem is connected to the thalamus and hypothalamus, as well as to higher brain structures and the cerebellum (see Figure A-1). It is divided into several parts. The lower part is referred to as the *medulla oblongata*. This inch-long section takes care of automatic responses like breathing, swallowing, and regulating blood pressure and body temperature. It works as part of the *autonomic nervous system*, coordinating with both cranial and peripheral nerves to induce involuntary, reflexive actions, such as causing the heart rate to increase or decrease, moving the diaphragm to regulate breathing, or creating "goose bumps" in response to being chilled or frightened. Other autonomic functions include the pupillary (relating to the pupils of the eyes) and swallowing reflexes.

Adjacent to and above the medulla is the *reticular activating system*, which is responsible for producing arousal and controlling sleep-wake cycles. The next landmark in the brain stem is the *pons*, which literally means the "bridge." It links the lower regions of the brain stem to the midbrain and the *cerebellum*. Complex interconnections of neurons occurring within the pons coordinate sophisticated motor movements of the body that require close regulation. With input from the cerebellum, the pons also helps maintain balance.

Passing through the pons, we find the *midbrain*, which is often divided into two parts containing structures involved with reflexive activity controlling both vision and hearing. These connections provide for the orientation of visual and auditory information with both eye and body movements so that we are able to effectively respond to external needs and threats. Its dorsal component contains the upward end of the reticular activating system and begins to process information both to and from the cerebellum. These parts govern most of the behavior that requires motor patterning to occur, such as eating, drinking, primitive grooming, and the fight-or-flight response.

Connected to these structures is the *cerebellum*. Cerebellum means "little brain." It is attached to the back of the brain stem, near the base of the skull, and has three lobes. The cerebellum coordinates all our movements, modulating, maintaining, and adjusting our every step, our every stance; it even coordinates the muscles that help us to speak. It also regulates the fluidity of speech by controlling the articulation of words and flow of sentences. Finally, it affects our ability to remember basic learned motor responses, such as riding a bike, responding to a handshake, or playing the guitar.

At the upper end of the brain stem, the midbrain connects with the *diencephalon,* the area of the brain consisting of the *thalamus,* which is the brain's relay center to the cerebral cortex, and the *hypothalamus.* The diencephalon mediates information from the brain stem to the limbic system and the cerebral cortex.

The *thalamus* and *hypothalamus* are the two all-important gateways to higher thought, emotion, and mental health. Every bit of information, every message, from the insignificant to the sublime, goes through the thalamus—a switching and relay system of sorts, much like the one at your local telephone company that matches a random incoming call with the appropriate outgoing line that will connect it with the correct number to complete the call.

A more human example is the connection you make with that great dress you saw in Macy's while rushing to work. That random impulse catches your attention, so it is sent to certain parts of your brain that can remember this fleeting event. At the same time, your emotions are heightened as you think about how you'll look at a party wearing that dress. These sensations are stored in your emotional brain, but the linkage is retained by the thalamic connection. When the occasion for such an outfit approaches, these connections will be recalled when you have time to go shopping. Only later in the process will more sophisticated areas of your brain become involved (one hopes) that will assess the cost of the dress in the context of your current circumstances. As these thoughts bounce from one part of the brain to another, the thalamus directs traffic, making sure that all bases are covered—from fit, color, and excitement to checkbook balance and ultimately pleasure. The executive functions of the neocortex balance all of these competing commitments in an attempt to prevent the long-term problems associated with pure impulse buying. This simplistic description of the thalamus and its major connections shows how important it is for your brain's higher functions to be in good working order— and how your thoughts and emotions can get confused, overwhelmed, and indecipherable when your brain is injured.

Right below the thalamus is the hypothalamus, one of the brain's control towers. Although no bigger than a pea, it's a dynamo of function. The hypothalamus controls eating patterns, sleeping and waking cycles, body temperature, blood sugar levels, emotional tone, sex drive, and hormonal (or chemical) balances. The hypothalamus also controls the *pituitary gland*—a major gland that regulates hormonal production and secretion. In other words, this small, pea-like part of the brain is responsible for maintaining the long-term internal stability of our bodies so that life remains possible. It governs vital functions and drives (activated in our brain stems) that keep us alive. It is also responsible for the control of the release of *cortisol,* a steroid that promotes healing when it is produced in the correct amounts at the right times—but if it is constantly produced, it evokes a chronic stress response throughout our bodies.

THE LIMBIC SYSTEM

The *limbic system* is a network of nerve cells that provides us with the capacity to feel; it supplies the emotional tone of our actions based on our memories and experiences. It has often been referred to as the biological basis of our emotional lives. We can feel anger, sadness, joy, and elation all as a result of activity occurring within the structures of our limbic systems. Because the limbic system is nestled right below the higher functioning cerebral parts of the brain, it ensures that emotions reach our conscious thoughts—and our thoughts affect our emotions. Both the limbic system and the cerebral cortex (that higher functioning part of the brain) actively influence each other. This helps to explain why events that are very emotional for us are so well remembered, whereas other experiences just float away with time.

It's easy to see how damage to the limbic system can affect a brain-injured person on a very intimate·level. Without emotion, or with inappropriate emotion, the patient may seem distant and disconnected from others. He or she may seem like a stranger to family and friends and vice versa if this area of the brain was affected.

The Hippocampus and the Amygdala

As very vital members of the limbic system, the *hippocampus* and the *amygdala* are responsible for much of what we remember and the tone of our emotions. The hippocampus looks like a sea horse and is located toward the front of the brain. It is directly connected to the senses—touch, sight, hearing, smell.

The hippocampus has the capacity to pick up the vision of a bright summer day and a flowery scent wafting on the breeze and to then connect this vision or scent with a memory of a similar summer day when you were a child, one it has stored for maybe twenty years. The hippocampus can then trigger the limbic system into action, evoking the emotion of nostalgia. And this emotion, in turn, helps to trigger the thinking areas of the brain—which will open the floodgates on the past and all the thoughts, promises, and long-ago dreams that the past implies.

This rush of memory and its emotional images are helped along by the amygdala, which sits in the middle of the limbic system. The amygdala plays a role in evoking a variety of emotional responses, but its size has been correlated with rebelliousness and, as you may imagine, is largest during adolescence.

However, there is more to thought than just emotion: Thought is the exercise of the mind in any of its higher functions, such as reflection, cogitation, learning, and judgment. These activities mainly occur in the cerebral cortex.

THE CEREBRAL HEMISPHERES

The two cerebral hemispheres together constitute the largest part of the central nervous system. This is what is commonly referred to as "the brain." The cerebral hemispheres are made up of neurons (nerve cells), glial cells, and other support structures, including blood vessels. Neurons have two parts, the cell bodies, or *nuclei,* which are gray, and their long connecting *fibers,* called *axons,* which appear to be white. The color of the axons comes from an insulating coat of myelin that facilitates electrical conduction from one nerve cell to the next. Thus, the grey matter is a vast collection of *nonmyelinated* neuronal nuclei, and the white matter is composed of bundles of myelinated axons and glial cells.

Although all mammals have cerebral hemispheres and a cerebral cortex, additions that are uniquely human are termed the *neocortex* ("new brain"). The neocortex contains structures that have evolved to the point of having highly specialized functions, not all of which can be tied to discrete areas contained within it. This is especially true of the prefrontal cortices, which are responsible for the *executive functions* involving reasoning and judgment. It is here that we organize and abstract, communicate and appreciate, create, perceive, and analyze—all those activities of thought and problem solving that make us uniquely human and distinguishable as individuals.

The executive functions come into play when we make conscious decisions. Once we have gathered all the data we can from talking with others, drawing on our past experiences, incorporating new learning, and infusing it with emotional tone, this external and internal information is ready for final processing. That final processing requires executive functioning and seems to rely heavily upon the front regions of both of our

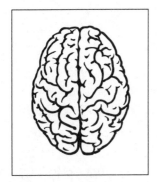

Figure A-2   The two hemispheres of the brain as seen from above

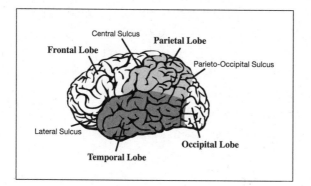

Figure A-3   The lobes of the brain

frontal lobes. Unfortunately, as we have seen, these areas are very vulnerable to injury due to their location within our skulls.

Like a patchwork quilt, the cerebral cortex is divided into halves and segments. Figure A-2 shows how clearly the halves can be seen.

Each half, called a hemisphere, is a mirror image of the other, and each consists of four segments called *lobes*. Each lobe has specific functions. Each one can be injured—and the injuries result in specific malfunctions.

THE LOBES OF THE CEREBRAL HEMISPHERES

Anatomists divide each of the cerebral hemispheres into lobes delineated by its most deeply extending convolutions, as shown in Figure A-3.

The Frontal Lobes

The frontal lobes are the "seats of power," the place where your personality anatomically exists and where it is created, honed, and refined with experience and maturity. These lobes supervise many activities and are responsible for the brain's executive functioning—from organizing to analyzing, from planning to decision making, from staying focused to perceiving what's in front of you. It is where the ego, your unique self that interacts with your surroundings, is housed.

If someone suffers damage to his frontal lobes, he will not be himself—literally. An injury there can affect everything from his ability to plan, understand an idea or a new situation, listen and pay attention, and keep his emotions in check to his ability to empathize, or see the world from a perspective other than his own, which forms the basis of intimacy and love. An injury of this type is therefore the most difficult of all to deal with emotionally, particularly for the patient's loved ones.

The Parietal Lobes

The parietal lobes are found between the frontal and occipital lobes and above the temporal lobes. Between the abutting areas of the parietal and frontal lobes are strong connections that involve muscle movement and sensations. These areas play an important role in bodily sensation, much in the same way the adjacent areas of the frontal lobes control motor movement, with each side governing the sensations or movements of the other side of the body (*contralateral*). Furthermore, they play an important role in reading, enabling the reader to bring letters together as words and turn words into thoughts. Injury here can create amnesia, abnormalities in sensation, and *neglect syndromes*, in which a person might not perceive that his left arm belongs to his body and neglect to bathe and dress it.

The Temporal Lobes

Next to the frontal lobes are the temporal lobes, which derive their name from the Latin word for "forming the sides." These lobes, located near the cheekbones, house the *auditory cortex*—a small area about the size of a quarter—which enables us to make sense out of what we hear. The lobes are also involved in certain perceptions and memories. Parts of the limbic system make up or are intimately connected with the temporal lobes. Damage to the temporal lobes can result in problems with comprehending language and speaking words that communicate meaningfully, deficits in working memory, and roller-coaster emotions.

The Occipital Lobes

Located in the back of the cerebral cortex, these lobes take in information from our eyes and analyze what we are seeing. Damage here can result in an unusual type of blindness known as *cortical blindness*. The eyes retain their ability to "see," but the occipital lobes do not know or recognize what they are functionally seeing. The eyes let other functioning parts of the brain know that something is "out there," but without the interpretative abilities of the occipital lobes we cannot process that information into useful knowledge of the object itself. One of my patients who had brain damage to his occipital lobes, for instance, was able to see an object to avoid walking into it but couldn't tell you what the object was.

ONE BRAIN, TWO HEMISPHERES

We've all heard people say things like "she's really right-brained," for a creative artist, or "he's really left-brained," for a computer whiz. These statements contain a grain of truth, but they can be a bit misleading. It is true that the two hemispheres are different, but they work in tandem, even if not completely in unison. Like Siamese twins, they share an organ and they look alike, but they don't quite talk, behave, or think alike.

In general, the left hemisphere controls logical thinking, language skills, and numerical calculations; it tends to control movement on the right side of the body. The right hemisphere is responsible for visual memories and the ability to make art, play music, or dance; it tends to control the movements of the left side of the body. The right side sees "the forest," the big picture down the road. The left side sees "the trees" and can connect the dots between each one and conceptualize their growth. If you injure the left side of your brain, it will affect the right side of your body; conversely, if you injure the right side of your brain, it will affect the left side of your body.

It is immediately noticeable just how much brain area is devoted to controlling parts of the body most associated with our humanness. For

The Essence of a Horse

One of the landmark studies of right-left brain behavior involved an artist who had his corpus callosum severed in an accident. When he used his right hand to draw a horse (which meant that his left brain was in charge), the drawing was perfect in every detail—save one. It was bookishly flat; it had no spark or artistic flair. However, when he used his left hand to draw the horse (which meant that his right brain was being used), he created a complete abstraction. Although this picture held no direct resemblance to a horse—no hooves, no tail, no mane—it was immediately identifiable as a horse because it held the essence, the soul of the animal, that was missing in the left-brain drawing.

example, in most people, even those who are left-handed, areas controlling speech and language are located on the left side of the brain. The right and left hemispheres work in tandem: The left brain gives a person the ability to speak, but the right brain gives speech its color, drama, and inflection.

Neglect syndromes occur with lesions on the right side of the brain in areas that organize bodily perception. Other functions of the CNS are not so clearly relegated to one or the other side. For example, executive functioning seems to be distributed throughout both sides of the anterior frontal lobes, although subtle differences, such as a tendency to depression or mania, have a greater likelihood of occurring when a particular side is lesioned—a left anterior lesion is associated more often with depression and a right anterior lesion with mania. Nevertheless, the two hemispheres are in constant communication with each other via a thick bridge of nerves called the *corpus callosum*. When this bridge is severed, the right and left sides each work independently, as if the other didn't exist.

Damage to any area of the brain, whether a hemisphere, lobe, or part of a lobe, can result in someone "not being himself," but A doesn't always lead directly to B. Like most relationships in life, it all comes down to communication.

The Nerve Cells, or Neurons

In order for bits of information to get from every part of the body to the parts of the central nervous system where they can be deciphered, understood, and acted on, they have to travel a convoluted path from the farthest parts of the body to the spinal cord and eventually to the brain. For example, if your finger touches a hot stove, the information has to travel from the finger to the hand and then up the arm via the peripheral nervous system. Then, it goes from the first part of the central nervous system—the spinal cord—where a reflexive action is immediately generated without input from higher brain structures. This communication very rapidly permits a response that will move your arm and hand away from the stove to prevent further damage to your finger.

However, the message doesn't stop there; it travels up the spinal cord to the brain stem and the thalamus, which directs it to the appropriate higher functioning areas of the brain. The sensation of instantaneous tissue damage will now become describable as pain. At this point, the message will move to various brain centers, from the limbic system and the hippocampus to the temporal lobe and on to the frontal lobe, and further be transmitted from the left hemisphere to the right and vice versa. Of course, all this must occur as every other vital function remains controlled and the body continues to send other data to the brain for processing.

The way the central nervous system sends messages is somewhat similar to the way we send e-mails through cyberspace via cable, satellite, or DSL. In the brain and the rest of the central nervous system, a network of signals and wires connects every part to every other part. These "wires" are nerve cells, or *neurons*. They carry messages using both electrical impulses and chemical conductors. They are shown schematically in Figure A-4.

An electrical impulse carries all the information from the beginning of the neuron, known as its dendrite, to its axonal tail. Some axons may be several feet long, such as those coming from the arms or legs. During this part of its journey, the message is transmitted electrically, which explains the high speeds of transmission discussed above. However, to ensure that these electrical impulses do not run amok, they are regulated. The regulation

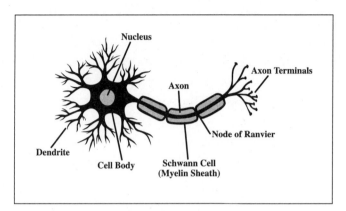

Figure A-3   The parts of a neuron

occurs at the axonal synapse, the space between the dendrite and the axon. The electrical energy of the axon must be translated into chemicals called *neurotransmitters,* which literally must be released from the *synaptic vesicle* and then move through a fluid-filled gap known as a *synapse.*

Think of a synapse as a river without a bridge and the neurotransmitters as the "boats" that carry the chemical energy to the next cell. If a sufficient "fleet" of neurotransmitters is released, they will permit the electrical discharge of the next neuron to take place, propagating the message electrically forward. The change back from a chemical signal to an electrical current occurs at the outlying *dendrite* tentacles of the next neuron, which may receive similar impulses from a number of nearby neurons.

The neurotransmitters themselves are silent until stimulated, "quietly" waiting like docked boats in *vesicles* (cell storage compartments) near the synapse. Only certain classes of neurotransmitters are capable of activating specific channels in the next cell by selectively binding to it, much as a key fits into a lock, opening a single door.

Although the messages themselves can pertain to everything from hunger to feeling cold, from worry to wonder, from decisions at an ATM to guilt about an overdue phone call, the basic theme is one of coordination and inhibition of competing, stimulating impulses. Furthermore, there is always feedback from the stimulated cell to the neuron that propagated the excitation.

One of the hallmarks of humanness is the ability to inhibit and control impulses until such a time occurs, if it ever does, when it is appropriate to gratify them. This is what permits humans to function in groups and form communities. Newer research has shown that a brain injury stimulates a cascade of inappropriately discharged excitatory neurotransmitters that have the ability to destroy living axons by permitting the entry of ions into those viable axons that eventually causes their cell walls to break down, leading to massive axonal degeneration. If this cascade could be interrupted, we would be able to limit the damage associated with both traumatic and acquired brain injuries. Unfortunately, the current interventions under study must be attempted within hours of the injury or they are ineffective.

Anatomy and physiology can only help us understand so much. Even as we pinpoint the various neurotransmitters and the electrical impulses sweeping throughout the brain, there is a part of each one of us that no one else sees, a part that cannot be fully understood by our expressed behaviors. It is the self—and it is bigger than the sum of all these processes combined.

RESOURCES

AMERICAN HEART ASSOCIATION
National Center
7272 Greenville Avenue
Dallas, TX 75231
800-AHA-USA
www.americanheart.org
Comprehensive source for information on all aspects of cardiovascular disease.

AMERICAN HEALTH ASSISTANCE FOUNDATION
22512 Gateway Center Drive
Clarksburg, Maryland 20871
800-437-2423 or 301-948-3244
Fax: 301-258-9454
www.ahaf.org
Information on scientific and medical investigations on stroke and heart disease.

AMERICAN STROKE ASSOCIATION
7272 Greenville Avenue
Dallas, Texas 75231
United States
1-888-4-STROKE
www.strokeassociation.org
Comprehensive source of information on strokes.

BRAIN ATTACK COALITION
31 Center Drive, MSC 2540
Building 31, Room 8A-16
Bethesda, Maryland 20892
301-496-5751
www.stroke-site.org
Dedicated to decreasing occurrence, disability, and death due to strokes.

BRAIN INJURY ASSOCIATION OF AMERICA
(Each state has its own chapter)
800-444-6443
www.biausa.org
Largest organization for information on TBI.

Example: Brain Injury Association of Georgia
Brain Injury Resource Foundation
1841 Montreal Road, Suite 220
Tucker, Georgia 30084
888-334-2424 or 678-937-1555
Fax: 678-937-1557
www.birf.info
Web site has worldwide database on brain injury information.

CENTERS FOR DISEASE CONTROL AND PREVENTION (CDC)

1600 Clifton Rd.
Atlanta, GA 30333
800-311-3435
www.cdc.gov
Fact sheets on TBI, strokes, and heart attacks.

DEFENSE AND VETERANS BRAIN INJURY CENTER

Building 1, Room B209
Walter Reed Army Medical Center
6900 Georgia Avenue NW
Washington, DC 20307-5001
800-870-9244
www.dvbic.org
Dedicated to TBI veterans and their families.

MEDLINEPLUS

U.S. National Library of Medicine
8600 Rockville Pike
Bethesda, MD 20894
http://medlineplus.gov
www.nlm.nih.gov
Web site devoted to providing information to help answer health questions by the National Institutes of Health.

NATIONAL INSTITUTES OF HEALTH

9000 Rockville Pike
Bethesda, Maryland 20892
www.nih.gov

National Institute on Disability and Rehabilitation Research (NIDRR)
www.ed.gov/about/offices/list/osers/nidrr/index.html
Educational support for research related to the rehabilitation of individuals with disabilities.

National Institute of Mental Health
Office of Communications
6001 Executive Boulevard, Room 8184, MSC 9663
Bethesda, MD 20892-9663

National Institute of Neurological Disorders and Stroke (NINDS)
P.O. Box 5801
Bethesda, MD 20824

National Library of Medicine
8600 Rockville Pike
Bethesda, MD 20894
http://medlineplus.gov
www.nlm.nih.gov
All have large databases of information on rehabilitation topics and disorders.

U.S. DEPARTMENT OF VETERANS AFFAIRS: REHABILITATION RESEARCH AND DEVELOPMENT SERVICE

Veterans Health Administration
Rehabilitation Research & Development Service
Washington, DC

Publications
103 South Gay Street, 5th floor
Baltimore, MD 21202
Information and journal on rehabilitation issues for veterans, but applicable to all groups.

ACKNOWLEDGMENTS

There are far too many individuals involved in the writing and production of a book to give adequate acknowledgment to all of them. Yet, I would like to express particular gratitude to Lee Woodruff, who gave her time and prodigious talents to writing the foreword to the book and sharing her family's personal experience with brain injury. I am also indebted to Joelle Delbourgo, my literary agent for providing the "glue" that put this project together in the first place and kept it going despite the inevitable bumps along the way. To Karla Dougherty, for helping to shape parts of the book, as well as introducing me to Joelle, which ultimately led to a contact with Da Capo Press and the opportunity to work with their very professional and talented staff. Further, to my editor Wendy Francis at Da Capo Press for believing in the book since its inception and for providing invaluable assistance in keeping the project advancing with her wealth of experience and knowledge in publishing. In addition, I wish to thank Carrie Cantor for her exceedingly critical assistance in scrutinizing every word of the text, thereby insuring that the work would be accessible to its intended audience.

INDEX